This Isn't Working

The Crisis of the Mental Health System and the Prescription It Needs

Natalie Kurkjian M.D.

To my father, who always told me to "write it down."

ACKNOWLEDGMENTS

David Hall, thank you for sharing your tact for writing, your willingness to let me keep the semi-colons, and your genuine interest and investment in making what I wrote better.

Christopher, for your persistent and unwavering support in making this happen.

My family, for encouragement I needed.

H and E, you were likely unaware that I peeled away at your bedtime to write this book. My hope is that one day you will also find the reason and conviction to "write it down."

Lastly, to my patients. Thank you for your trust and willingness to let me enter your lives.

Preface

"Why did you choose psychiatry?"

I am a practicing psychiatrist, and I am asked this question multiple times a week. By nurses during my clinical rotations in medical school, by new acquaintances, by my patients, and by my colleagues. And yet, for how often I'm asked this question, I always hesitate. It's such a natural thing to ask someone why they chose their career, but with psychiatry, it is surprisingly difficult to answer simply.

And I'm sure every psychiatrist will tell you something different. My best answer on why I became a psychiatrist is that I feel mental health obfuscates and complicates every other issue, whether we're talking big societal stakes...or the day-to-day struggles of the individual. When I look at the discourse of our society, mental health issues are clouding the picture. It's the fog. It is, to me, the loud, annoying beep in a silent room. And it is affecting *everything*.

Case in point: someone I will never forget, and I hope you won't, either. Picture a woman, early 30's. Her bleached-blonde hair has recently become unkempt. We'll call her Lisa. She had been admitted to the university hospital where I was a third-year medical student on my internal medicine rotation, not for any psychiatric issues, but for uncontrolled hypothyroidism and type 2 diabetes. Lisa had prescriptions for both conditions, but she was not following the medication regimen. Making her treatment doubly difficult for her physician, Lisa, clearly exhausted, could be combative and frankly abrasive in discussions about her treatment. For some background, thyroid hormones affect many parts of your body's functioning. From a mental health standpoint, too much thyroid hormone can make someone extremely anxious, on edge, and in extreme cases, even psychotic. Too little can make someone apathetic, depressed. She was my patient and part of my daily rounds. One morning, in the gentlest way I could approach her, I tried to "lift the veil." I used what my professors had taught, including the power of silence, and given the chance, she answered the questions I asked. She shared about struggling financially, and how at one point she was rationing her medications because she had to use her disability money that month for her child, who was having difficulty with school and needed a tutor. She talked about being depressed and not wanting to get out of bed, leading to her not taking her medications for her thyroid and diabetes. As is so often the case, mental health issues had become one more major obstacle in getting a patient well.

This case, one of many, was the reason I went into psychiatry. Psychiatry allowed me to focus on a piece that seemed to be missing from effective medical care, the mental health piece. I wanted to "lift the veil." I wanted, and still want, to clear the fog. And over time, I found out that not only did I like doing it, but I was also good at it. I could help a patient feel at ease, and that to me was more than what I could offer in other fields of medicine.

Lisa is one of millions. Millions of people with mental health issues, with some getting the treatment they need, some falling through the cracks in the system and receiving inadequate care, and others shambling through without the treatment they need, surviving day to day with serious disadvantages and risks. According to the 2019 National Survey on Drug Use and Health, nearly 20 million adults in this country went through a major depressive episode that year (World Health Organization, 2019).And that was before a major pandemic. That is 20 million people who need a mental health care system that is working; *our mental health care system isn't working.*

So where do I exist in this system?

I am a board-certified psychiatrist. This means I passed an 8-hour board certification exam after I completed my four-year psychiatry residency on top of four years of medical school. Since then, I have continued to fulfil requirements of the psychiatry board to continue my certification. I see patients both "in clinic," also known as an ambulatory outpatient clinic, and in the medical hospital setting. Those in the latter category have already been admitted into the hospital and are experiencing psychiatric issues that require my expertise. I see patients in various settings, and so I treat patients in different levels of care.

So why write a book about the mental health system?

Even in my relatively short career, I have come up against countless fixable areas that hinder the care any person in this society can receive or does receive. They could affect whether you even have access to a psychiatrist when you need one. Even if you do get in with a psychiatrist, the hiccups to your care may not end there. The entire American health care system is a constant political topic that usually ends with some conversation on how it can be "fixed", but I assure you, the mental health care system specifically is much more fragile. The delicate conversations that exist in every area of our society around the "mental health" of a person signal an anxiety about the system. Our society is uncomfortable with mental health. Discomfort breeds inadequacy. In this book we will touch on system shortages, insurance issues, and other roadblocks to one receiving adequate care.

For now, let's start with the basics, in particular the need for psychiatric health care. Wait times to see a psychiatrist can vary from 4 weeks up to 6 months. If you are looking for a child and adolescent psychiatrist, especially one who takes insurance, or Medicaid, that wait could be even longer. That is four to six months a person must potentially wait with no treatment beyond what their general practitioner or an urgent care facility or emergency department will provide. That's not a sign of a healthy or robust system working. Just think: your average episode of depression can remit within 6 months, if treated with medication and/or therapy. In the time it takes for a potential new patient to see a psychiatrist for the first time, they could have already undergone treatment and put the whole situation behind them!

And what can happen to a potential patient while they're waiting for their treatment? The risk of suicide is what immediately comes to mind when we're talking about mental health issues. However, there are more insidious risks associated with inadequate mental health care. According to the World Health Organization, there is a 10-20 year reduction in life expectancy for those living with a severe mental disorder like moderate-to-severe depression (Fiorillo & Sartorius, 2021). Like in Lisa's case, simple self-care becomes more difficult, and the patient's overall condition worsens. So, while the worst-case scenario in health care is loss of life, what is also important to mention in the field of psychiatry is the *quality* of life that is lost. This loss may not be unique to psychiatry and mental health. But while the patient with hypertension is untreated and waiting for treatment to take effect, they may not feel well. But "not feeling well" in psychiatry has wide, strong ripples. Loss of employment, family structure, financial difficulties, to name a few. Accessing psychiatric care is the start of this conversation. We'll explore this more in the next chapters.

And that's the clinic side of mental health. What about the mental health issues in the medical hospital setting? Just ask the nurses. There's a certain moment when I turn the corner walking out of the elevator, and I start to make my way down the hallway to the medical ward. After several years of employment, the nurses, social workers, and case managers have learned the time of day when I tend to round on patients. By nature, when the hospital staff see a white coat descending the hallway, they tend to poke their heads out to see if that white coat is relevant to their needs. But having observed this phenomenon for a while now, I would attest there is a different atmosphere when I make my way towards them. They see me coming down the hall, and often the nurses ask hopefully, "oh, you're going to room 431, right?" or "You must be heading to room 323!" Their hope is explained by the fact that often an uncontrolled psychiatric issue in the medical hospital yields a more complicated hospital stay, often marred by patient discomfort and physical and emotional distress for any family or healthcare worker.

In the hospital setting, the same facts of the outpatient world hold true. Again: if you address the mental health issue that may be complicating other factors, the overall situation will improve. So, if a patient is admitted with a urinary tract infection that has been allowed to fester and has now become delirious, which can cause a patient to become uncharacteristically physically agitated, the overall care of this patient has reached a higher level of complexity. Complexity, in health care, equals more time, more money, and more personal effort. These three corners make up a significant portion of areas of focus for health care reform.

Try to imagine a hospital, full of trained professionals moving through its halls like determined ants through an anthill—dedicated people tougher than the 12-hour shift, and each with more medical knowledge in their heads than people a hundred years ago could have dreamed of—and imagine that rock-solid institution being worn down, not by an epidemic of germs, but an unrelenting parade of mental health issues. If this sounds a little scary to you, good.

Imagine how it feels to *be there*.

This is a problem we can solve. Or, perhaps more realistically, if not solve, *MAKE BETTER*. Put another way, we may not be able to cure the condition, but we can treat it. What it will take, at this stage, is knowledge, discussion, and creation and utilization of resources.

Mental health. When a physician documents in the chart, they utilize the basic structure learned in medical school. The SOAP note. Subjective, objective, assessment, and plan. What did the patient say to you, what does the data say, what is your assessment, and what are you going to do about it? We'll utilize this structure in a way to address many facets plaguing this system. I think of the Albert Einstein quote: "If I had an hour to solve a problem, I'd spend 55 minutes thinking about the problem and 5 minutes thinking about solutions." (Sturt & Nordstrom, 2013). To solve the problem, you must know the problem.

You're about to see the world of mental health in a way that normally takes 8 years of school and 4 of residency. And all you had to do was open this book.

Who is this book for? In short, this book is for you. In an existential tone, you is anyone and everyone who wants to understand the mental health crisis. This is for those in healthcare, those who are not in healthcare, those in politics, healthcare policy, or basically anyone who cares about, has been affected by, or is currently struggling with their mental health care.

Mental health, behavioral health, psychiatry, psychology. It's what matters. It affects every little thing. There is not a field of medicine it does not affect. Going further, there is no other field of medicine where outcomes could not be significantly improved if mental health were part of the treatment. For example, recent research revealed that of the thousands of veterans with a mental health condition who were subsequently diagnosed and treated for lung cancer within the VA (Veterans Affairs) health system lived longer if the veteran also received concomitant mental health treatment (Berchuck et al., 2020).

So, I invite you to follow along for the next few chapters as I touch on some of the most important subjects I think anyone on this planet needs to know and understand about mental health. It'll be educational, hopefully interesting, and at least shed some light on the crisis of mental health we are in and what could be expected.

To begin, we'll start with who makes up the mental health team. Next, we'll look at many administrative and resource roadblocks that prevent or slow the advancement of mental health care. Finally, we'll glance at a few clinical issues which are even now affecting millions of people. Every aspect of the mental health system and its ailments could be its own book. As a person on the inside, I hope to share what I have seen and what we can expect to see in the future.

Why did you choose psychiatry?

Initially, I chose it to help people. And we have so many people to help. By effectively evaluating and meeting the challenges of this broken system, we can save millions of people's lives (not to mention billions of dollars in wasted medical spending!)

Of note, the book has examples of clinical cases. These cases were taken from medical journal articles, news articles and other open-source resources. Some clinical cases were inspired by patient cases from my residency training, including patient cases presented by residency colleagues. All details of the patients have been changed to protect privacy. There is one exception. One patient from my residency training did give consent for her case to be written. She was extremely proud of the changes she made. Her details were still changed to protect her privacy, but if she ever reads this, she'll know this is about her and I know that will make her happy.

Let's get started.

Berchuck, J. E., Meyer, C. S., Zhang, N., Berchuck, C. M., Trivedi, N. N., Cohen, B., & Wang, S. (2020). Association of Mental Health Treatment With Outcomes for US Veterans Diagnosed With Non-Small Cell Lung Cancer. *JAMA Oncol, 6*(7), 1055-1062. doi:10.1001/jamaoncol.2020.1466

Fiorillo, A., & Sartorius, N. (2021). Mortality gap and physical comorbidity of people with severe mental disorders: the public health scandal. *Annals of General Psychiatry, 20*(1), 1-5.

Sturt, D., & Nordstrom, T. (2013). Are You Asking The Right Question? Retrieved from https://www.forbes.com/sites/davidsturt/2013/10/18/are-you-asking-the-right-question/?sh=64ea76a376c5

World Health Organization. (2019). Premature death among people with severe mental disorders. *https://www.samhsa.gov/data/sites/default/files/reports/rpt29393/2019NSDUHFFRPDFWHTML/2019NSDUHFFR090120.htm#:~:text=Among%20the%2019.4%20million%20adults,year%20from%202009%20through%202018.*

Chapter One

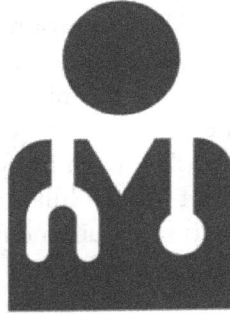

The Mental Health Team: Who They Are and Where They Came From

We've all had the experience of sitting in the waiting room, patiently twiddling our thumbs, or browsing mindlessly on our devices, while we wait for the doctor's assistant to call us in. Whether you were waiting to see your psychiatrist, your primary care physician, or a specialist physician, some of the same thoughts probably crossed your mind: *I wonder what the doctor is doing right now? Will she know what's wrong? Will she be able to help me?*

By the time your appointment is over, you will hopefully have answers to most of these questions, but you've probably never had an answer to the first one: *What is the doctor doing right now?* No, your doctor is not sitting at the desk, feet propped, sipping warm coffee, and eating bon-bons, watching clinic get backed up by 10 minutes, 20 minutes...Your doctor is actually asking him or herself questions all about you! And clicking endlessly on various check boxes on the digital chart to fulfill government and insurance documentation requirements.

What questions is your doctor asking? *What is bringing this patient in? What could be causing the issue? Does the patient need labs or imaging completed to get to an answer?* Answering these questions, for the physician, begins before she ever lays eyes on you. The physician's well-trained mind is like a large, complex engine, and it is already turning over, activating years of training and experience. And the physician's mind is working very quickly, as more patients are being checked in for their appointments.

But, as our healthcare system has become more complex, an increasing number of these questions have become of a non-medical nature. Questions like: *Will the patient be able to afford the medications I prescribe? Will insurance cover their medications? If I need to refer them to a specialist, how long will it be till they are seen?*

And back in the waiting room one of the most impactful questions in healthcare is being asked -- *can I trust my doctor?*

The trust between a physician and patient is even more substantial in the field of psychiatry. After all, why *should* the patient trust the physician? What are our qualifications?

Let's get to it.

Whether they're your primary care physician, your dermatologist, your heart surgeon or your psychiatrist, your doctor has given up years of their life to earn the privilege of treating you. These are *intense* years. Only those who truly love medicine can expect to make it. My own medical school class had 160 students. This is a little smaller than normal. Some classes number less than a hundred, but most classes today are generally a few hundred strong (Powell & Kowarski, 2021). Of those 160 students in my class, only 8 went on to specialize in psychiatry.

Finding your specialty is a little, well, intense, life-changing, speed-dating. Move over, Tinder. The process to pick a specialty and then choose a residency predated the "swipe-right" of current online dating. As a third-year medical student, you're lifted from the quiet, safe classroom, where your patients are just examples given in textbooks, and assigned to what's called *clinical rotations*. It's just like it sounds. You're literally rotated through different clinical positions, normally for a few weeks at a time. At each rotation, you practice real medicine "in the field." Always under close supervision of an attending physician, of course.

More specifics.

Clinical rotations are a huge part of an aspiring doctor's training. He or she will be in clinical rotations for, generally, two years of medical school. Core clinical rotations, usually including general surgery, Ob-Gyn, internal medicine, family medicine, pediatrics, and psychiatry are completed in the third year. Each rotation is a full-time job, with shifts lasting between 12 and ideally, 24 hours. The exposure to various facets and environments of each specialty exists so that each medical student, near the end of the 3rd year, can choose their specialty with confidence. Confidence that based on a mere few weeks of experience, they will dedicate their life's work to that specialty. It is quite a commitment. To pick a specialty, one must know themselves, their capabilities, and then imagine a life-long career in that specialty. Cue the most intense swipe right.

In psychiatry, rotations may be completed in a psychiatric inpatient setting, an intensive outpatient program, a community mental health clinic, or in the medical ward of a hospital in the form of psychiatry consults. The psychiatry rotation is generally 4 to 8 weeks.

Medical school provides the foundation, but the majority of specialized medical education comes after graduation: enter *residency*.

What is residency? If you watch *Grey's Anatomy* or any medical sitcom, you might have the gist, although in real life there's no one off-screen keeping our hair perfectly messy or romanticized call rooms that any resident wishes to spend more than the necessary time in. This is a doctor's medical training *after* their medical training. A residency can last anywhere from 3 years (for, say, internal medicine) to 7 years (for neurosurgery) (American Medical Association, 2012-2013). Many physicians will testify that this on-the-job training is what will carry them through the rest of their careers. What lies before them is several more months of clinical rotations, all relevant to their specialty. Many rotations are outside the specialty to provide an all-encompassing education to the overlapped medical conditions that exist. Who decides what rotations a resident physician needs to experience? The Accreditation Council for Graduate Medical Education (ACGME) is a non-profit private council that oversees training for all physicians after medical school graduation. For each specialty, ACGME sets requirements for exposure to ensure each resident physician has completed necessary hours treating enough patients in different environments so that this physician can have the foundational knowledge and skills to start a career. For psychiatry residents, training in internal medicine and neurology is required by the ACGME (American Medical Association, 2012-2013). Internal medicine training for the psychiatrist is integral for understanding basic pathological conditions like hypertension, diabetes, thyroid disease, to name a few. These conditions are relevant in psychiatric patients. For example, the psychiatrist treating the patient with Attention Deficit and Hyperactivity Disorder (ADHD) with a mixed amphetamine salt stimulant, like Adderall, should know the risk of hypertension or cardiac adverse effects of these medications and feel comfortable treating the patient safely and appropriately (Sichilima, 2009). Second generation antipsychotics are notorious for causing metabolic syndrome. Specifically, they can increase blood sugar levels, cholesterol, and triglycerides in the blood. Awareness and understanding of endocrinology, often a rotation for psychiatry residents, provides not only exposure to diabetes but also thyroid conditions, which can often be misdiagnosed or mimic psychiatric conditions. Neurology is also required for psychiatry residents. While psychiatry looks at the emotional brain, neurological conditions often result in psychiatric conditions- such as stroke and depression but can also mimic each other. For some patients, seizures may not actually be seizures, but a psychiatric condition of pseudoseizures, or non-epileptic seizures, often resulting from severe stress. Neurology and psychiatry are closely related fields. In fact, they are even certified by the same board: the American Board of Psychiatry and Neurology.

Psychiatric residency lasts four years. During that time, after those foundational early months, psychiatry residents clock almost uncountable hours in psychiatric inpatient units, substance abuse clinics, child and adolescent psychiatric clinics, adult outpatient clinics, and cramming in varying levels of exposure to other areas in psychiatry as well. We cover many fields of focus, including forensic psychiatry, geriatric psychiatry, interventional psychiatry (electroconvulsive therapy, or ECT, eating disorders, and consult and liaison psychiatry, which we will get more into in another chapter. These rotations are supplemented with a diverse curriculum of classes that include psychopharmacology and psychotherapy training.

So, we discussed the training the future psychiatrist receives. What about the psychiatric training for the non-psychiatrist? As stated, the psychiatrist is exposed to internal medicine, endocrinology, neurology. Are these specialties in reverse exposed to psychiatry?

For most physicians, that initial psychiatry rotation in their third year of medical school will be the last time they are exposed to the undistilled psychiatric aspect of practicing medicine. For example, my father, who completed a residency in urology, had his last dedicated psychiatry clinical experience during medical school. So, do urology and psychiatry ever overlap clinically? Let's look at a diagnosis of interstitial cystitis (IC); IC is a chronic disorder of the lower urinary tract with primary symptoms of bladder pain with urinary frequency and urgency (Bendrick, 2022). It can be debilitating for patients. In the literature and clinically, patients with IC have been noted to have comorbid post-traumatic stress disorder (PTSD). Does the urology resident need to spend 4 weeks in a psychiatry rotation to know about this condition, its psychiatric component, and potential treatment? Logistically, no. But should psychiatry professors visit urology residents for teaching sessions? Probably.

Let's look at primary care physicians. Most primary care physicians have completed either a family medicine or internal medicine residency. How much psychiatry is in these residencies? The truth is the answer widely varies. In a simple data survey I completed during my residency training of family medicine and internal medicine residency programs across the country, I found there were several programs which had no psychiatric rotations at all for residents entering primary care. Other programs had a mere month of "Behavioral Sciences" as a rotation. While many programs highlighted their psychiatry rotations and the continued education in psychiatry, for the majority of programs viewed, the training is, simply put, just not enough. Not enough for the need.

According to one article, in the span of 12 years, prior to the COVID-19 pandemic, the proportion of primary care visits that addressed a mental health issue increased by almost 50% (Rotenstein LS, 2023).

How could a one-month rotation, in all the months (36 to be specific for family medicine) of a physician's training, prepare her for something she'll encounter in, presumably, a majority of her clinic visits?

How integral is the primary care physician to the mental health team? They are the spoke of the wheel, and often it is their evaluation, treatment, and referral that places a patient in a psychiatrist's office. I remember seeing this repeatedly in my medical school training.

During my primary care rotation, I was jarred by how often mental health was a significant factor in my supervising doctor's visits. I was rotating with a well-known, thorough, and most importantly, personable primary-care physician. She knew her patients, and vice versa. Her clinic had a strong sense of community, and with each visit, I could tell how much these patients appreciated their doctor. And for so many of her patients, she was treating a mental health issue, or were asking for referrals for said issue. Or, like Lisa, the woman with hyperthyroidism I introduced in the preface, they had a mental health issue that was acting as a catalyst for other medical problems. Of course, in those cases any immediate life-threatening issues had to be addressed first, and mental health issues had to be addressed later.

Let me share with you an experience from that time. It was a Friday afternoon, and the appointment was a last-minute add-on—a slot which the doctor usually saved for urgent needs. The patient was a young man, let's call him Andrew, around 19 years old, complaining of abdominal pain. Part of my training during this rotation was visiting with the patient to obtain an initial history and start documentation. I would then present this information to the doctor. For Andrew, I did as I had done all day. I listened dutifully as the patient and his mother related his trouble with abdominal pain, wrote down his history, gave them the good old "the doctor will be with you shortly," and took this information back.

That history I took down? Not relevant.

The doctor and I walked back in together, and the patient immediately broke down into tears. *Not* from pain. He was experiencing mild abdominal pain, but there was a much bigger issue. There had been a serious road accident a few weeks prior. Andrew, physically, was not significantly injured. But mentally, he was not okay. Ever since, Andrew had suffered such crippling anxiety riding in any car that he could barely tolerate that day's trip to the clinic. Fearing they had nowhere to turn, his desperate mother had called the doctor's clinic and embellished the abdominal pain to be seen. Why? I'm not sure as I did not ask. But I can imagine on that Friday afternoon, weeks having passed since the accident, as a mother desperate for her son to feel better, she turned to a physician who had helped them before. And so it fell to my supervising physician to change gears from considering abdominal pain and the need for imaging to anxiety and the need for immediate support and treatment. I recall leaving the patient's room walking side by side with the supervising physician. I turned to her, mouthing "Where did that come from?" She turned to me, knowing I had chosen a career in psychiatry at that point, and uttered, quietly, but in her usual colorful way, "Girl, you are so needed."

In fact, not only are psychiatrists needed—a whole team is needed to handle our country's mental health issues. Many people are aware of the relationship between doctors and nurses, and of how absolutely vital nurses are in treating patients' physical ailments. They're aware that nurses draw upon their own considerable reservoir of training. But people are often unaware that there are many more people delivering care than just doctors and nurses. All of them have specialized training important to keeping you healthy. To have a full understanding of the mental health industry as we pull back the veil, you'll need a working knowledge of all the players involved.

Meet the team.

On the more medical side of mental health care, there is the *advanced practice provider/clinician* (APP or APC) or referred to as a physician extender. APP are usually two different types of providers. There is the APRN, which stands for *advanced practice registered nurse*, AKA a nurse practitioner. This is a nurse who has completed extra schooling and clinical experience. In mental health, the APRN should have completed extra training and passed a certification demonstrating their clinical knowledge in psychiatry. Next up is the PA, which stands for *physician assistant*. This is a professional who has completed clinical training in various areas of medicine but usually has a focus in just one. We will talk a little more about this group and their roles in mental health in the coming chapters.

On the mental health side, let's talk about the people who put the patient "on the couch."

Traditionally, the professionals conducting therapy that places a patient on a couch are psychoanalysts. Historically, psychoanalysts were often physicians, but this has changed significantly towards psychologists, and other professionally trained therapists. Psychoanalysis certification requires extensive knowledge and practice of the pillars of psychological theory that explain "why does a person behave that way?" Think Sigmund Freud.

There's a wide variety of professionals patients may end up engaging in talk therapy, or counseling. They probably won't be psychiatrists, as changing tides of reimbursement and training has geared psychiatrists more toward medical management. The therapist, or counselor, may have a variety of letters following their names.

Licensed therapists come from a variety of educational backgrounds. They cannot prescribe medication (that's reserved for doctors, physician's assistants, nurses, and in some states, psychologists) but are critical in maintaining good mental health. Many mental health conditions can be ameliorated or even cured by therapy. Furthermore, licensed therapists are much more immediately accessible than your average psychiatrist. Let's do a brief rundown of licensed therapists. Each of these professionals not only has a master's degree but put in *thousands* of supervised clinical hours before they could be licensed to practice. The exact number varies by state, but it's most typically at least 3,000 hours within two years.

Remember, before we begin, that although a licensed therapist's educational background may give them some weight in a certain area, they each are capable of working with a patient across a wide range of areas. For instance, if a patient is looking for a therapist who specializes in trauma, the right fit could have LPC, LCSW, or PhD next to their name.

First, we have the LPC, or *licensed professional counselor*. This is someone with a master's degree in the straightforwardly named discipline of counseling. LMFTs, or *licensed marital and family therapists*, also hold a master's in counseling, but their work is more targeted on—you guessed it—married couples and families. LCSWs, or *licensed clinical social workers*, hold their master's in social work. While originally geared towards finding resources, LCSWs are increasingly more trained in different therapy modalities. Last, we come to the LADC, or *licensed alcohol and drug counselor*. The LADC has her master's in behavioral science and uses that knowledge to help you break self-destructive cycles (Caldwell, 2018).

A quick note about that last one: It's a common belief that the United States currently has a wealth of well-trained substance abuse counselors. But unfortunately, it's not true. And it's not getting better, either. In fact, the U.S. Health Resources and Services Administration (HRSA) has predicted that the country will experience a shortage of this critical personnel resource in the 2020s (Health Resources & Services Administration, 2013). What's more, LADCs are hardly the only mental health professionals we may be hurting for in the coming years.

Let's finish off this chapter by putting the spotlight on the psychiatrist's cousin: the psychologist.

It's easy for people to get these two categories, psychiatrist and psychologist, MD and PhD, confused. In an article by Dr. Torie Sepah about her time as a chief psychiatrist for the California Institution for Women, she relates her discovery that her own administrative assistant had been typing out Dr. Sepah's name on official documents with a "PhD." When she corrected her assistant that she was an "MD," she pointed out that "MD" was literally beside her name on her office door. The assistant said she'd thought Dr. Sepah was a not a medical physician, but a doctor like a psychologist, and that the door sign was a mistake (Torie, 2018).

As opposed to a physician's MD or DO, a psychologist's doctorate is either a PhD, or PsyD, which is basically a route to a doctorate that's less-research heavy and more focused on application and services to clients. Earning your PhD takes between 5 and 7 *years*. Psychologists, like other therapists, may focus on an area of psychology for their clinical expertise. Marital counseling, psychoanalysis, trauma-focused therapy, forensics. The expert who testifies that a person is not guilty by reason of insanity? Probably a psychologist. You'll see psychologists in all facets of the mental health system. They are integral to research development and clinical treatment.

So clearly, we have a wide variety of therapists, counselors, and psychiatrists, a team of mental health professionals ready to help you in your greatest time of need. But a difficult question arises for many patients when you need help: *Can you reach us?* Or rather, can you reach the mental health care you need in general? The truth is, it's getting more difficult for average Americans to get access to the care they need.

In the next chapter, we'll focus on the hurdles patients face in getting, and even *keeping*, care.

Your ground-level education is complete. You know all the players. It's time we started pulling back the veil and diving into the serious problems plaguing our mental health care system.

American Medical Association (Producer). (2012-2013). Graduate Medical Education Directory Retrieved from https://www.acgme.org/globalassets/PDFs/2012-13.pdf

Bendrick, T. R., Sitenga, G. L., Booth, C., Sacco, M. P., Erie, C., Anderson, D. J., Kaye, A. D., & Urits, I. (2022). The Implications of Mental Health and Trauma in Interstitial Cystitis. *Health psychology research, 10*(4), 40321.

Caldwell, B. (2018). *Basics of California Law for LMFTs, LPCCs, and LCSWs (fifth edition)*.

Health Resources & Services Administration. (2013). *Health Workforce Projections: Addiction Counselors*. https://bhw.hrsa.gov/data-research/projecting-health-workforce-supply-demand.

Powell, F., & Kowarski, I. (2021). 10 Medical Schools With the Most Students. Retrieved from https://www.usnews.com/education/best-graduate-schools/top-medical-schools/slideshows/10-medical-schools-with-the-most-students

Rotenstein LS, E. S., Landon BE. (2023). Adult Primary Care Physician Visits Increasingly Address Mental Health Concerns. *Health Affairs*, 163-171.

Sichilima, T., & Rieder, M. J. (2009). Adderall and cardiovascular risk: A therapeutic dilemma., *14*(3), 193–195.

Torie, S. (2018). How psychiatrists became lesser physicians. Retrieved from https://www.kevinmd.com/2018/02/psychiatrists-became-lesser-physicians.html

Chapter Two

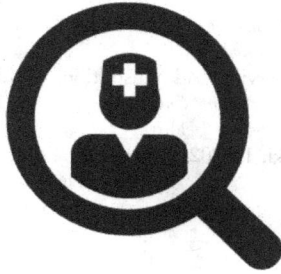

Access to Care and Insurance

The Doctor Will See You Now

Research has shown that anywhere from 30-70% of primary care visits are mental health related. This means if you start to experience debilitating anxiety or mood issues, which are some of the most common chief complaints seen in the primary care setting, you will likely first be seen by your primary care physician (PCP) or clinician (APRN, PA). Further, psychiatrists will often require a referral to their clinic, usually from the primary care physician or clinician--especially if your PCP is employed by a hospital system.

I had a friend once ask me for help finding care for their nephew. The child's pediatrician recommended he see a child and adolescent psychiatrist for an evaluation and treatment. The parents were given a list of possible referrals, but due to prolonged wait times, they wanted to see if I knew of other options. I gently responded that finding mental health care is a full-time job that no one wants to apply for. Let's understand why. Meet Mr. B.

Mr. B is a 32-year-old gentleman with no past psychiatric history. Yet he has started to notice some new concerning issues. He cannot seem to sleep well. He experiences racing thoughts, especially at night. He has found it difficult to go to work, and in fact, has called into work for sick leave three times in the last three weeks. He has started to isolate himself from friends and family. This has been going on for almost four weeks. His family has noticed and encouraged him to seek help. He makes a new patient appointment with his family medicine physician, Dr. L.

It's standard practice guidelines for a general medical visit to screen for depression and anxiety. Screening tools, like the PHQ-9 and GAD-7, have been validated by several clinical studies showing that by using these scales, symptoms of depression and anxiety can be captured for diagnosis and ultimately treatment (Kroenke, 2010). Let's say that Mr. B's responses resulted in scores meeting criteria for depression and anxiety. Dr. L sees these results, discusses options with Mr. B which include starting treatment then and/or a referral to specialists, namely a psychiatrist and therapist for treatment of both conditions. Mr. B opts to start treatment and asks that a referral is placed for both a psychiatrist and therapist.

Let's pause.

From here, we're going to examine an *ideal* journey into psychiatric access, one where everything works as it's supposed to. In this land, care is delivered urgently, insurance covers all evaluations and treatment, and the patient has the time and financial opportunities to commit to these evaluations and treatment.

Before Mr. B leaves, Dr. L places a referral in his own clinic network. For clarification, Dr. L is not a solo practitioner, working alone in a clinic. Dr. L works for a large health system marked by a vast network of primary care physicians, specialty physicians, and surgeons of all disciplines. While the referral is being processed (insurance authorization) behind the scenes, Dr. L discusses the treatment that can be initiated while the referral is making its way to a psychiatrist. Mr. B agrees and Dr. L prescribes Mr. B an antidepressant. This antidepressant will take 4-6 weeks to take effect. He tells Mr. B that a scheduler from the psychiatrist's office will soon contact him to schedule his first appointment. Until then, Dr. L encourages Mr. B to practice good sleep hygiene, watch his diet, and to get some fresh air and exercise every day. Mr. B leaves the clinic with a prescription sent to his pharmacy and a follow-up visit on Dr. L's schedule in 4 weeks. This visit is scheduled because Dr. L knows his health system psychiatrists are scheduling patients anywhere from 1-4 months from the time of the referral.

So this is ideal. Even this simple story doesn't usually go this way. First, the assumption that Mr. B could swiftly get in with a PCP is a bit of a reach. Oftentimes, a patient may have to wait 1-2 weeks or longer to establish care with a PCP. So that's not too terrible.

But the referral to the psychiatrist. Mr. B happened to go to Dr. L who works for a healthcare system. What this means is there is a health system, for illustration we will call it Cardinal Health System. So, this Cardinal Health System employs Dr. L. Besides Dr. L, who is one of many primary care physicians in the system, this health system also employs four psychotherapists and three psychiatrists. Again, this is ideal. So, this referral goes to what is often called the Behavioral Health clinic.

Here is where things get more complicated. Stay with me.

Mr. B has an insurance called, again for illustration and not reality, Hummingbird Health Insurance. His referral is received at the Behavioral Health clinic. In an ideal situation, the psychiatrists are "in-network" with Hummingbird Health Insurance. This means there has been an agreement between Hummingbird Health Insurance and the psychiatrist. The psychiatrist has been credentialed through Hummingbird Health Insurance and this insurance will pay for the services Mr. B needs. But I said it got more complicated.

Let's say Hummingbird Health Insurance decided they did not want to cover behavioral health needs. So, they contract with what is called a "carve out" insurance, like a secondary insurance, for mental health coverage. This insurance is called Black Crow Insurance.

Mr. B starts to go through the intake process (insurance, screening questions) for the behavioral health clinic, but this time, he is told the psychiatrists in the behavioral health clinic are not "in network" with Black Crow Insurance. Our Mr. B is about to become Mr. 0, as in zero dollars to his name, because he's about to pay out-of-pocket at the full rate. If Mr. B wishes to use his insurance, he will have to hunt for a psychiatrist with a different hospital system covered by the Black Crow insurance network.

Does he have options? Sure. He could try to appeal to his insurance to cover "out of network benefits," as in pay at least some of these services. But more often than not, Mr. B will simply be quoted the high prices he would have to pay since his insurance is not in network. Imagine Mr. B's confusion. Imagine asking why you're fine to see Dr. L, who works in the same hospital system as the psychiatrists, but you're now being told your insurance is out of network? Both doctors working under the same roof, and yet one is covered by your insurance, and one is not!

Imagine bringing a gift card to Target or some other department store, but your card is only good for items in certain departments—and you don't realize which until it's time to check out!

Welcome to the first hiccup in seeing a psychiatrist. Insurance, access, and coverage of services.

Mr. B at some point opted for Hummingbird Health Insurance through the government marketplace for insurance plan purchase. And as a 30-

something year-old man with no history of psychiatric issues, he realizes later, or when it matters, as above, that Hummingbird Health Insurance has mental health coverage, as it is considered an essential health benefit for marketplace insurances and many others ("Health Benefits and Coverage," 2023). But the devil is in the details.

While mental health and substance abuse coverage is considered an "essential health benefit", understanding what will be covered, to what extent, and for how long is integral to one receiving the care they need to return to a previous level of functioning. Otherwise, a person with mental health needs and inadequate treatment is hopping from train to train hoping to reach their destination. Twenty-five years ago, Mr. B's insurance may not have covered his behavioral health care. Or if they did, the insurance may not have covered his behavioral health care at the equal level, also referred to as parity, as his medical coverage. For example, prior to the parity legislature, Mr. B may have paid a $25 copay for seeing his PCP but would have a $50 copay for seeing a psychiatrist. Mental Health parity laws have appeared several times, most recently in 2008, with the Mental Health Parity and Addiction Equity Act of 2008 (Pestaina, 2022). While the parity legislature has the best intentions, unfortunately it does not apply to all health insurances, and often mental health clinicians are categorized as "specialists", as in not your general practitioner, so the copay may be higher.

Let's revisit the moment Dr. L's assistant gave a list of psychiatry referrals to Mr. B. There was one group we skipped over: the psychiatrist who does not take insurance. Let's understand this group better.

Around the 1990's, insurance companies decided to change how they were paying psychiatrists. They began to favor the shorter 15-minute medication check, checking the patient's response to the medication regimen, over the longer, 45 or 60-minute traditional therapy session. What came from this, naturally, is that psychiatrists followed suit and leaned toward the shorter "med check." But what also happened is that many psychiatrists stopped taking insurance *entirely*. The patient has the option to file for out-of-network benefits, with responsibility usually resting on the patient to file it with their insurance to see if their insurance would pay, well, anything. A simple flat rate for new patients and follow-up patients started to emerge.

So back to our Mr. B. He is not dealing with the above issues, both because he lives in an idyllic hypothetical scenario, and also because he opted to see physicians working for a health system. Not taking insurance is not an option due to the *employed physician* element. Mr. B's doctor does not, on his own, have the power to make the decision to accept or reject insurance. According to his employed physician contract, that power lies with the health system he works for. And of course, all major hospitals take insurance. However, the potential for roadblocks still exists. For instance: just how many psychiatrists are even out there for Mr. B to see?

In the introduction, we discussed data on the dwindling number of practicing psychiatrists in the United States, and now it's time for the data to speak.

The average wait time to see a psychiatrist, as a new patient, is 3-6 months. That is 90 days. This unfortunate state of affairs affects various people differently. For instance, if someone is starting to feel depressed, it is possible the depression can resolve itself, if mild, with improved sleep, rest, exercise, good nutrition, in those 90 days. Of course, for many, resolving an episode of depression in 90 days is a conservative estimate.

Before I continue, I want to note there are available resources for those who are needing assistance sooner. There are essentially 3-4 levels of care available for those with mental health needs. Outpatient care (see psychiatrist in clinic) is considered the lowest level of care. Above this, there are intensive outpatient programs (abbreviated to IOP), then partial hospitalization programs (PHP) that afford more intense monitoring, medication adjustments, and support. Psychiatric hospitalization is the highest level of care and considered to be the mainstay of treatment for those in crisis. I don't think you'd be surprised to know that yes, your health insurance matters significantly for these options. The state mental health systems, funded by taxpayers, create access for anyone with any financial situation to have emergent psychiatric care. But for the in-between, the IOP or PHP programs will require insurance authorization for acceptance and length of the program. For example, the program for an IOP consists of multiple sessions of group therapy on multiple days of the week. This is in addition to psychiatric medication management, either by a psychiatrist or APP. Other supportive programs like art therapy are included in daily programming. So, if Mr. B is declining while he is waiting to see a psychiatrist, Dr. L can direct Mr. B to an IOP or PHP, for a higher level of care. And guess what process starts over- where can Mr. B go and for how long?

But what can be done to increase access to care?

Let me introduce the collaborative care model (CoCM). Enter the AIMS (Advancing Integrated Mental Health Solutions) Center at the University of Washington. They created a model, that is in use at this time, to change the usual general physician-to-psychiatrist referral.

In the collaborative care model, Mr. B would see Dr. L in clinic, as before. Mr. B would be screened for depression and anxiety. Dr. L would then add Mr. B to a list of patients who are being screened and managed for depression and anxiety. Then, on a previously scheduled day, Dr. L would meet with a Behavioral Health Care Manager, who collaborates between Dr. L and Dr. P, a psychiatrist who practices in a city 100 miles away. This care manager would collect the data Dr. L has on Mr. B regarding his scores for depression and anxiety, and take this information to Dr. P, the psychiatrist, who would then review this information. Dr. P would give recommendations regarding a medication regimen. This information is then given back to Dr. L by the case manager. Hence, there is a collaboration.

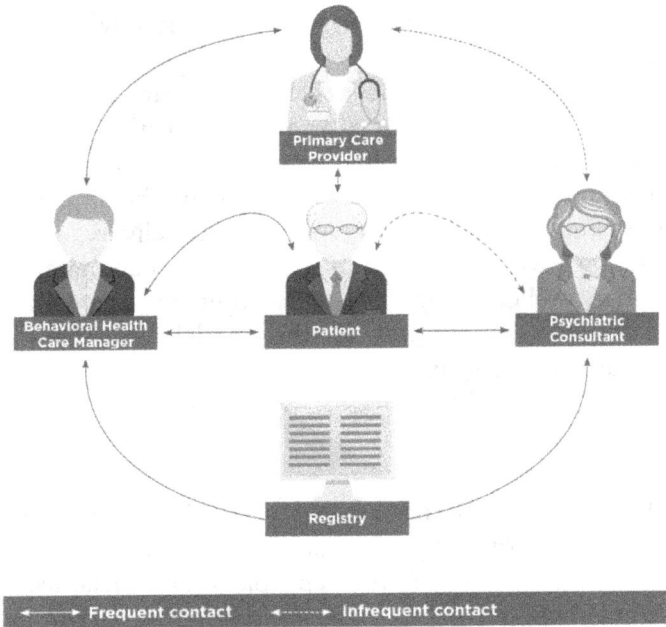

(American Psychiatric Association, 2023)

Since its inception in the 1990's, the CoCM has developed into an evidence-based practice. More than 90 randomized controlled trials and several meta-analyses have demonstrated the CoCM to be more effective than typical treatment for many common behavioral health diagnoses, including depression and anxiety ("Collaborative Care," 2023).

Another model used is that a psychiatrist is housed in the primary care setting. So, a clinic which has 5-6 general physicians, one psychiatrist is available for immediate consults or evaluations. If a patient scores high on the PHQ-9 or GAD-7, they are ushered to the psychiatrist on the same day for an outpatient consultation.

In my opinion, the collaborative care model is currently filling the care gap that exists within mental health care. The collaborative care model for treatment was supported substantially by the approval of billing codes for this type of care delivery; thus, insurance will pay for this care which eliminates a barrier. Whether by third-party companies or within health systems, we will see this model more widely available in the near future.

Prior Authorizations

This next element affecting the care of mental health patients is not unique to the field of mental health care. I guarantee if you approach any healthcare provider who works in the outpatient clinic setting and mention the words "prior authorization," their eyes will not be able to roll far enough back in their head. Cue the eye rolling emoji.

Prior authorization (what clinic personnel often shorten to a "prior auth' or just 'PA'), to sum it up briefly, is when the insurance company requires that there is an authorization, essentially a clearance, given from the company before proceeding with any intervention a medical clinician is recommending. It could be surgery, medication, or even just a preventative measure. The clinic and physician must have prior authorization from the insurance company if the patient wants the action to be covered (most often in my case, this is a medication prescribed to a patient).

I'll give you three guesses why this is the case. Money or cost are most often cited as reasons a medication must have a prior authorization. Another reason? Necessity. The insurance company can insist that the medication may not be actually necessary for this patient and alternatives must be considered. By withholding coverage in this way, the insurance company can actually *override* your doctor's recommendations for your treatment.

As mentioned, you can probably deduce how physicians feel about this process. Physicians, tired and weary, carrying hundreds of thousands of dollars in student education debt, just want to deliver good health care. And for many, any barrier between you and your doctor's recommended course of action is met with hostility. But before I tear into this concept, let's be fair and consider that there are a handful of constructive outcomes tied to prior authorization.

For instance, and I will build more on this later, but direct to consumer marketing of medications has become especially problematic. I'm talking about those medicines you see in TV commercials, where an attractive person with perfectly styled hair and a sensible sweater is looking out the window and sighing discontentedly. Then (like magic!) the filter which has been muting the colors of the attractive person's world is peeled away, and they are now at a barbecue in the sunshine, with radiating positivity and hope for the future. Just ask your doctor if this person can be you.

In psychiatry in particular, these medications are usually costly, and are targeted at a very small population. But because of their cost, pharmaceutical companies will bypass physicians and target patients/consumers directly with expensively produced advertising. This is not to say doctors are completely cut out of the loop. Clinicians are courted with paid lunches or gifts to entice the medication to be purchased. Cue dollar sign emoji.

So, let's see this in action. A patient enters their psychiatrist's office, is screened for, and diagnosed with depression. The patient requests the $1400 per month medication they saw on TV that is intended for patients with a diagnosis of bipolar disorder. The psychiatrist's first response is to counsel the patient that the medication they are asking about is FDA-approved for bipolar disorder and using it to treat simple depression is what's considered off-label use (without FDA approval but research has shown to have positive outcomes). If the patient still wishes to try the medication off-label, the psychiatrist will offer to order the medication but will advise that the insurance company may require a prior authorization, and the medication may not be approved. If your insurance does not approve the medication for off-label use, then obviously you can still pay for it, but your insurance won't cover it.

Often, the desired medication is not approved, and cheaper alternatives or medications intended for that diagnosis are suggested.

This is just one of the many clashes of pharmaceutical company versus insurance company, with the actual clinician who is sitting with the patient stuck in the middle. In this case, the insurance company is trying to be mindful of medications that are more likely to be beneficial and/or more cost-prohibitive to the patient.

But apart from this scenario, prior authorizations are under much scrutiny. They require considerable administrative time. If the clinician is lucky enough to have clinic support to help fill out the multiple questions required, a fair chunk of time will be saved. But even then, the documentation needed to attest to the requirements for this patient can cause considerable strain on the functionality of the clinic and even the mental health of the clinician.

Let's talk concrete examples. In residency, I remember one of my first experiences with prior authorizations. I had a patient who had been stable on a medication for two years. But the insurance company decided they wanted a prior authorization for her refill she requested. The clinic medical assistant filled out most of the form, leaving one section for me to fill out.

It asked the following: "What medications previously did the patient take for this condition?"

On this day, I relied heavily on my frontal lobe to exercise the impulse control necessary to keep me from writing, "The same freaking medication the patient has been stable on for two years. Are you kidding me?" (Honestly, I wanted to use different words, but I don't want this book to take a different direction).

Where are we in medicine that we require of a success, a patient who is medically stable on a medication, a minimum of an extra of 30 minutes to prove to the insurance company that their medication is necessary? This patient's stability on this medication likely saved their insurance company countless dollars while the patient did not require the emergency room or psychiatric hospitalization for two years. But in their computer algorithms, or whatever labyrinthine systems they have, that day, a prior authorization was needed. Luckily, I had outstanding clinic assistance, so these prior authorizations and refill requests were handled in a timely manner. When problems arise, it is typically because the insurance company and pharmacy cannot reach an understanding; or, we have filed an appeal because, often, with my expertise I feel I must advocate for what medication is best for my patient. Usually in the latter situation, I'll prescribe an alternative to help the patient as much as possible while we await the results of the appeal. My clinic is lucky to have the resources to handle the added burden of prior authorizations. But not all clinics are as fortunate. So, who suffers when a clinic cannot handle the extra burden the insurance companies are placing on it? The patient, of course.

In July 2022, an article exploring the case of Kathleen Valentini, who died waiting for a prior authorization, was shared widely on medical news sites and the media. "Did a prior authorization delay kill Kathleen Valentini?" was the sensational, yet not hyperbolic, headline.

The background of this patient is as follows: Valentini was experiencing hip pain. She sought medical care and followed their recommendations, but the pain did not remit. Her physician thought the next step was to pursue further imaging, specifically an MRI, as a simple X-ray had not shown any cause for the pain. But Valentini's insurance required a prior authorization before it would cover the MRI. Her physician made her case to the insurance company, but it was ultimately denied, a decision that would have tragic consequences. But who made this fateful judgement? Behind the scenes, it is now known her health insurance company uses a 3rd party company to review prior authorizations for any patient insured.

The prior authorization denial stated that Valentini should pursue physical therapy —which, in fact, she had already completed. This process of requesting prior authorization, followed by denial (complete with a useless recommendation), followed by appeal, caused a delay of 40 days before Valentini could have her doctor-recommended MRI. It showed what no one wants to see. She had sarcoma, aka cancer of bone and soft tissue. Further testing showed metastatic cancer in her lung. Her physicians advised that had the cancer been discovered sooner, Valentini could have been treated with chemotherapy and possibly more localized surgery. Instead, she required amputation of her leg, hip, and pelvis. Despite these drastic measures, Valentini ultimately died two years later (Gallegos, 2022).

So why does this health insurance company, whose existence is predicated on financially safeguarding you from costly medical care, decide what is medically necessary? When did trained physicians lose critical decision-making power to mysterious third-party advisors?

While this case is on the far end of the spectrum of severity, it can be presumed that along that spectrum, there are multitudes of cases where a patient's health is allowed to worsen, or a condition is allowed to deteriorate, or simply that a patient's symptoms are not adequately treated, because an insurance company (or undisclosed third-party company) decides that this patient does not merit the doctor-recommended intervention.

Virtual Sanity or Insanity?

The 1996 hit "Virtual Insanity" by the UK band Jamiroquai, widely remembered for its futuristic music video but also cautionary message against virtual ubiquitousness taking over reality, had the following lyrics (Jay Kay, Stuart Zender, Derrick McKenzie, & Buchanan, 1996).

Futures made of virtual insanity, now
Always seem to be governed by this
love we have
For these useless, twisting, of our new
technology
Oh, now there is no sound, for we all
live underground, wow

As mentioned, virtual care has instrumentally and forever changed the landscape of medical care. Out of the most trying medical time in a generation, the COVID-19 pandemic, few developments in the health community compared to the fast and widespread use of "telehealth." Deregulations of requirements for use of telehealth allowed medical care for individuals across the country to continue remotely. Several of these suspended regulations had limited the care that could be delivered through virtual means. One example is the regulation that states a clinician must only see a patient in the state where the clinician holds a medical license. So, is that a problem?

I should probably give more background here. A physician's medical degree is not a free pass to practice medicine anywhere in the country. A physician actually also has several licenses and certifications. Licenses allow the physician to practice in the state in which the license was issued. If you live in West Virginia but wish to live in California for 3 months of the year and practice medicine while there, you must have applied, completed all requirements, and hold an active license for California. This strict licensing requirement changed with the pandemic. If you lived in Texas but wanted to see a patient who lived in Colorado, this was now possible. Other regulations exist regarding where the patient can be physically seen, besides what state they live in. Virtual check-ups, for instance, were not covered by insurance prior to the pandemic. Also, for those insured by Medicare, the government acknowledged the fact that not all patients will have access to a smartphone with audio/video capabilities, or even have internet access at home. So, during the height of the pandemic, Medicare allowed for audio-only visits to be conducted. And to ensure continued care for those under Medicare, CMS (Centers for Medicare and Medicaid Services) pushed for equal payments for these visits as for those completed in-person. This also allowed the older and more vulnerable population to stay home for their medical care and reduce their risk of contracting COVID-19.

Seeing my patients where they live, even just through a computer screen, has allowed them to share their lives very viscerally with me in ways I could not have imagined before the pandemic.

I have had the privilege of being taken on tours of their homes. Several patients have shared art projects with me that were keeping them busy during quarantine. I have met just so many adorable dogs and cats, although many of the latter appear to believe it is their right to be the star of their owners' laptop screen.

Other situations created by telehealth visits have been less constructive. Certainly, privacy has been more of an issue. I've learned to ask if anyone else is present for the visit, out of sight of the laptop or phone camera, and ensure the patient wishes for that person or persons to be present for the appointment. But other obstacles have also cropped up. Safe driving and proper dress code, to name a few.

But this is not the only example of the pandemic spurring a good policy decision that's also had some ill effects. Let's talk about the Ryan Haight Act, formally the Ryan Haight Online Pharmacy Consumer Protection Act of 2008. Enforced by the Drug Enforcement Agency (DEA), this Act holds rules regarding the prescribing of controlled substances by telepsychiatry. This legislation was literally created in the name of patient safety regarding medications that can be addictive and/or dangerous if consumed in large amounts. A critical component of this Act requires an in-person evaluation of a patient within a certain interval of time to ensure proper management and supervision of the patient receiving the medication ("Ryan Haight Online Pharmacy Consumer Protection Act of 2008," 2023). With the COVID-19 pandemic making routine in-person visits dangerous for both patient and doctor, this rule was wisely suspended. For clinicians like me, the suspension of this rule has been instrumental in allowing me to continue seeing patients virtually, even as we've left the worst of the pandemic behind us.

But with all good things comes those who take advantage, am I right?

Within a short time of the suspension of the Ryan Haight Act, several startup companies appeared to fill the gap for those needing psychiatric care. Sounds fine, right? It wasn't.

In May 2022, the US Department of Justice initiated an investigation of the mental health startup Cerebral due to prescriptions of medications Xanax and Adderall, used for the treatment of anxiety and ADHD, respectively. The following month, CBS News released its own report on the company and its practices. They found patients had an easy time acquiring medication but struggled to get into contact with their prescribers later, leading to adverse outcomes. After the announcement of the investigation by the DOJ into their practices, Cerebral stopped prescribing Xanax and Adderall (Livingston & Dodge, 2022; Werner & Kegu, 2022). So, has the pendulum swung too far, the door been opened too wide? It's worth a discussion. Perhaps the most important angle we need to answer this question is: how does this situation affect patients? We want everyone to have access to the medication they need, even if they can't regularly physically attend sessions with a psychiatrist at a clinic. But whether it's in-person or telehealth, maybe a full session must be the guide rail for psychiatric prescriptions. Consider: According to the Association of Nurse

Practitioners, the typical caseload for nurse practitioners dispensing psychiatric medication is 15 patients per day. But according to nurse practitioners formerly employed at Cerebral, they were seeing twice that number at 30 patients a day. That comes out to four patients an hour. Any company which is known to be "pressuring providers to dispense drugs after too-brief virtual sessions" is not just a risk for patients, which is more than enough to discount the "care" they provide, but a possible drain on public money as taxpayer-funded facilities pick up the pieces for Cerebral's struggling customers (Mosendz & Melby, 2022). While the mental health crisis is apparent, rashly providing care without measuring the quality of care could yield actual less savings or improvement than before.

The suspension of the Ryan Haight Act and other regulations over telehealth and telepsychiatry have resumed to some degree. But the American Psychiatric Association, among countless others, are approaching the government to consider continued suspension and even amending of these regulations to continue virtual care. Telehealth has created incredible avenues of quality care for psychiatric patients, but the policy isn't just a train switch, locking the tracks in one direction or another. We must proceed thoughtfully and with moderation as we find the right balance to provide the best care for patients.

American Psychiatric Association (Producer). (2023, 11/6/2023). Learn About the Collaborative Care Model. Retrieved from https://www.psychiatry.org/psychiatrists/practice/professio nal-interests/integrated-care/learn

Collaborative Care. (2023). *University of Washington.* Retrieved from https://aims.uw.edu/collaborative-care

Gallegos, A. (Producer). (2022, July 1). Insurer Delays Prior Authorization, Patient Loses Leg and Pelvis, Then Dies. *Medscape.* Retrieved from https://www.medscape.com/viewarticle/976486

Health Benefits and Coverage. (2023). *HealthCare.gov.* Retrieved from https://www.healthcare.gov/coverage/mental-health-substance-abuse-coverage/#:~:text=Mental%20and%20behavioral%20health %20services,and%20behavioral%20health%20inpatient%20s ervices

Jay Kay, Stuart Zender, Derrick McKenzie, & Buchanan, W. (1996). Virtual Insanity. On *Travelling Without Moving.*

Kroenke, K. e. a. (2010). The Patient Health Questionnaire Somatic, Anxiety, and Depressive Symptom Scales: a systematic review. *General hospital psychiatry, 32, 4,* 345-359.

Livingston, S., & Dodge, B. (Producer). (2022, May 16). Leaked email: Mental-health startup Cerebral will stop prescribing most controlled drugs like Xanax and Adderall. *Business Insider.* Retrieved from https://www.businessinsider.com/cerebral-to-stop-prescribing-most-controlled-substances-2022-5

Mosendz, P., & Melby, C. (Producer). (2022, March 11). ADHD Drugs Are Convenient To Get Online. Maybe Too Convenient. *Bloomberg.* Retrieved from https://www.bloomberg.com/news/features/2022-03-11/cerebral-app-over-prescribed-adhd-meds-ex-employees-say#:~:text=Seven%20former%20nurses%20for%20the,fueli ng%20a%20new%20addiction%20crisis.

Pestaina, K. (Producer). (2022, August 18). Mental Health Parity at a Crossroads. *KFF.* Retrieved from https://www.kff.org/private-insurance/issue-brief/mental-health-parity-at-a-crossroads/

Ryan Haight Online Pharmacy Consumer Protection Act of 2008. (2023). *American Psychiatric Association.* Retrieved from https://www.psychiatry.org/psychiatrists/practice/telepsychi atry/toolkit/ryan-haight-act

Werner, A., & Kegu, J. (Producer). (2022, June 22). Former Cerebral employees say company's practices put patients at risk: "It's chaotic. It's confusing. It could be extremely dangerous". *CBS*

News. Retrieved from https://www.cbsnews.com/news/cerebral-ceo-mental-health-startup/

Chapter Three

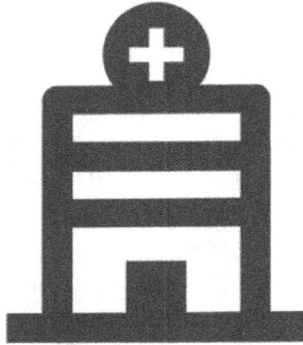

Geraldo Rivera

Yes, you read that title correctly. This chapter starts with Geraldo Rivera, television reporter and media personality.

In early 1972, Rivera was an investigative journalist for a local TV station in New York City. Finding egress through a back door, Rivera entered the Willowbrook State School on Staten Island with a film crew in tow. This school housed nearly 6,000 intellectually disabled children and adolescents. Its capacity was only 4,000.

Rivera had received a tip about the school's conditions. He started an investigation. One thing led to another, and Geraldo Rivera found himself documenting a facility crammed with children and adolescents in a horrible state of neglect. In an environment where patients outnumbered caretakers 50 to 1, children in dire need of daily aid were left almost to fend for themselves. Rivera was shocked to find children malnourished, sometimes without clothes, some even left to play in their own feces. But the problems even went beyond heartbreaking neglect; he uncovered physical and sexual abuse of the residents by staff of the school (Rivera, 1972).

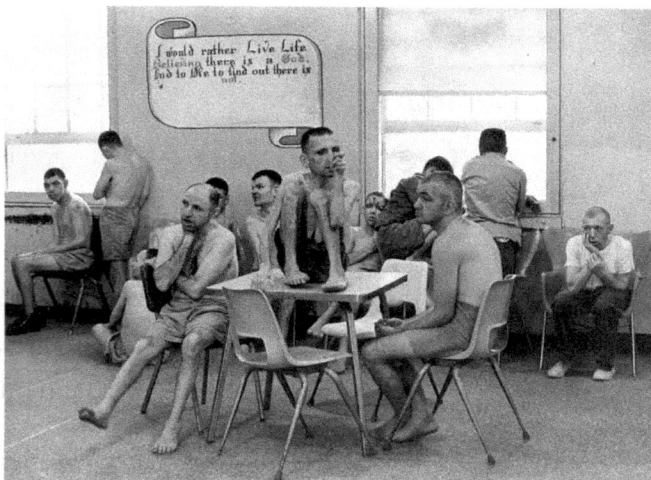

(Disability Justice, 2022)

Rivera's resulting exposé, *Willowbrook: The Last Great Disgrace* won a Peabody Award and forever changed how America looked at long-term institutions for the mentally disabled.

A class-action suit was filed against the state of New York by parents of residents in 1972.(Disability Justice, 2022) The school eventually closed in 1987.

In February 2020, *The New York Times* did a follow-up report of where the residents of Willowbrook had landed (Weiser, 2020). Most of the residents ended up in group homes. Group homes can best be described as a home managed by caregivers with residents living in a typical "house" setting, instead of a facility. Often 3-6 residents live in a house, depending on the size of the home and the number of caregivers.

Unfortunately, the *Times* investigation uncovered still more mistreatment of the school's alumni after they had left. In 2019 alone, ninety-seven reported allegations of physical abuse by group home workers against alumni were noted. There were also further allegations of abuse, neglect, improper use of restraints or seclusion, medical errors, and theft.

So why am I sharing these tragic stories with you? What am I hoping you'll take from all this?

Let me share some more background.

One Flew Over the Cuckoo's Nest. If you have not read this classic American book, you may have seen its adaptation, famously featuring Jack Nicholson. If you've seen the movie, the stark white walls and general sense of the milieu in which the patients lived probably comes to mind.

The institutions depicted in *Cuckoo's Nest* did exist, as shown by Willowbrook. However, in the time since these works were released, the concept of psychiatric hospitalization has evolved dramatically. There are still artifacts from older models, especially in state-funded hospitals where patients may stay long-term. Most psychiatric hospitals, however, are what's called *acute care hospitals*. What this means is, say someone has a crisis. And say this crisis is an urgent psychiatric need, usually severe depression with suicidal thoughts, drug or alcohol problems, psychosis, or bipolar disorder. This acute care need is treated in a psychiatric facility with an average length of stay of around 3-10 days. Oftentimes the length of stay is influenced by the opinion of the patient's insurance on how long they should stay, but a discharge usually depends on the patient's mental status and stability.

Willowbrook State School was the old model. While this model was geared more towards those with intellectual disability, the concept of someone with a mental health issue being "institutionalized" has fallen out of favor. And from the reports, even besides those stemming from Rivera's work at Willowbrook, for good reason.

But this begs the question: if institutionalization is out of favor, and hospitals are attuned to acute care needs, then where does someone with a serious mental health issue or developmental disability go for long-term care if there is no one to care for them?

For SMI (serious mental illness) including severe schizophrenia or bipolar disorder, this often means jail, prison, the department of corrections. According to a state survey completed by Torrey, *et* al. approximately 20 percent of inmates in jails and 15 percent of inmates in state prisons have a serious mental illness. At the time of the survey (2014), the approximated number of patients with SMI living in state hospitals was 35,000. This number compared to the approximated number of 356,000 inmates with SMI living in jails and state prisons, with less-than-optimal psychiatric treatment, is a testament of this problem. (Torrey & Zdanowicz, 2014).

Outside of these diagnoses, the staggering statistics surrounding autism demonstrates a rapidly growing issue. In 2020, the CDC estimated an increase in autism prevalence by nearly 10 percent, to 1 in 54 children in the U.S (Autism Speaks, 2020). Approximately 1 in 3 children with autism are considered more severe, marked by low IQ, difficulty with speech, and an inability to fully care for themselves (Zeliadt, 2019). Severely autistic patients may also display aggressive, even violent behavior towards themselves and others. This can make taking care of them, especially with younger family members in the house who may be at risk of injury, difficult. There is a dearth of resources available to help people care for children and family members with severe autism. And with the shortage of child psychiatrists, at-home care becomes even tougher.

I present two patient cases. One case was inspired by a case reported during a residency training lecture. The other was derived from a case report. Again, as always, facts have been adjusted for patient privacy.

Callie is a 32-year-old woman with severe borderline personality disorder who resides independently. She is *followed*, or closely managed in other words, by a community mental health clinic

PACT worker (Patient Aligned Care Team) who comes to her apartment nearly every day to administer her medications.

But unfortunately, Callie is not always home. The reason why has to do with a manifestation of her BPD that's relatively unknown outside of medical circles. Many BPD patients enact self-harm such as "cutting." In Callie's case, her self-harm manifests as "deliberate foreign body ingestion"—literally, swallowing non-nutritive and harmful objects. If you monitor her medical chart at one facility and review shared information from other facilities in the area, you would see Callie visits an ER 4-6 times a week, each time after swallowing another object--often a pen, a fork, or even a knife.

It was reported on one occasion that, as Callie was signing out AMA ("against medical advice," which is her routine when she wants to leave to smoke a cigarette or she is growing frustrated by being in the hospital), that she swallowed the pen she was using to sign the papers. Although she wanted to leave the hospital and had demonstrated at that time the capacity to make that decision, she reportedly became so emotionally charged in that moment, that she impulsively swallowed the nearby pen.

What caused this behavior? Callie has a very severe trauma history, stemming from her childhood years in foster care. The fewer details given about the nature of her trauma, I feel, the better.

On another occasion when she was being evaluated, a nurse asked a question which you yourself are likely asking: "Shouldn't she go to a psychiatric facility?"

Well, I believe she should. As concerned as people are about abuses that can occur at long-term psychiatric care facilities, the truth is institutions of the stripe of Willowbrook and *Cuckoo's Nest* are fifty years in the past. Today's institutions are vastly preferable to leaving Callie alone to fight a losing battle against harming herself. But as to whether she *can* go to such a facility? Despite Callie's clear need, seeing her admitted is a difficult proposition. She first must be accepted. And by this point, after several years of this behavior, every single facility in the state knows her. And knows that not much will come out of accepting her but an eventual transfer to an emergency room after she manages to swallow something. Psychiatric facilities are not urgent care facilities, and patients with unstable or chronic physical conditions needing treatment more invasive than, say, oral antibiotics cannot be housed in a psychiatric facility.

Callie's supervision needs are relatively high. Most psychiatric facilities simply don't have the staff to constantly watch her one-to-one, which is extremely important. Most psychiatric facilities simply will not have the resources to remove the high-risk inedible objects she swallows. Each time Callie, who is remarkably resourceful, got her hands on something inedible to swallow, she would need to be shuttled to an acute care hospital for removal. As noted, this could be happening half a dozen times a week, or nearly every day, constantly disrupting any constructive psychiatric treatment, not to mention severely draining financial support and staff away from other patients.

What Callie probably needs is electroconvulsive therapy- aka shock treatment. Despite what you may have seen in *Cuckoo's Nest*, it can have a profound beneficial response on those with severe mental illness. But I digress.

The reason I've presented Callie here is to highlight a unique, albeit rare, case of serious mental illness that has no great option. She has mental health services coming directly to her apartment, but even then, her safety is not guaranteed. So where should Callie go?

She is estranged from her family. No acute care inpatient psychiatric facility will take her. And even if they did, it would be a short-term hospitalization, likely shorter than normal in her case due to her history of ingestion.

There is a difficult question we need to ask when considering patients like Callie. When the "institutionalization" of mental health patients was regarded as inhumane and mental health patients were placed in alternative facilities or worse, released with limited resources into the community, did the pendulum swing too far?

Should the homeless mental health patient with limited resources end up in jail for small crimes? Or should he be placed safely in a long-term facility where he can receive medications and treatment that can lessen his symptoms? Should he have resources be available where he could actually work a job and feel he has purpose?

My next case is Randall. Randall is also 32 years old. He has severe autism. He is verbal but has a vocabulary of maybe 100 words. He has extreme outbursts, and has broken many pieces of furniture, and unintentionally harmed his mother and brother. The family is supported by the state. His mother was employed but had to stop working because of Randall's severe autism. His brother cannot work because he needs to be home to help care for Randall, especially to manage his severe outbursts. He was in a state-run facility for 2 years because of the severity of his illness and the state's opinion that Randall was not being cared for at home.

His mother alleges that possible abuse happened while Randall was in the care of the state.

This family is struggling. They find joy in little moments, but the lives of Randall's brother and mother are frozen by his severe autism. They are not alone.

I have encountered patients with various levels of intellectual disability. Some of my patients have been fortunate, like Randall, and are cared for by loved ones at home. In these cases, the caregiver is usually supported financially by the state. This situation, while difficult for the caregiver ("caregiver burnout" is a common and documented issue), is what I think could be considered ideal.

Another consideration for care options is a group home. An outside agency contracts and provides staff to care for 3-4 patients in an actual home, outfitted to serve those with intellectual disabilities. As the realities of COVID-19 and relaxed telehealth regulations moved outpatient care to virtual appointments, I have been afforded the opportunity to see a patient of mine who lives in a group home. I have worked with the patient's caregiver for several years. He is kind, attentive, and my patient does not look distressed and appears well-taken care of. That is the hope.

Roadblocks

During my residency training, I recall visiting with a patient in the emergency room who needed to be transferred to a psychiatric facility. The hospital where I did my training did not have its own psychiatric floor or attached psychiatric hospital. The most the hospital could offer was a social worker, assigned to psychiatric patients in the emergency room, who would fax their paperwork to multiple psychiatric facilities around the state hoping to find a bed.

"Find a bed. Find any bed."

Ask any emergency room physician in this country how they feel when they read those sentences. I have zero doubt you would hear a groan, see an eye roll, and possibly a full body shudder. This is because, in this country, we have a bed problem.

I'm not talking whether the mattress sold by sheep is better for sleep or the environment. I am referring to the urgent need for psychiatric inpatient beds.

In 2020, the American Psychiatric Association created the Presidential Task Force on Assessment of Psychiatric Bed Needs in the United States. 42 doctors and therapists collaborated on a 131-page report that was published in May of 2022, titled "The Psychiatric Bed Crisis in the US: Understanding the Problem and Moving Toward Solutions." (American Psychiatric Association, 2022)

In the report, the authors looked extensively at the current, historical, and future trends regarding inpatient psychiatric treatment. What they found was what every psychiatrist had already seen: a considerable decrease in bed availability from the 1960's to today.

What is the cause? While the authors do discuss how treatment modalities have changed since the 60's, the paper assigns greater blame to the effect of "managed care." That is, how have insurance companies changed the psychiatric inpatient bed landscape? As we mentioned earlier, the process of being admitted to a psychiatric hospital drastically changed as insurance companies took a leading role in deciding a patient's appropriate or necessary treatment. So, hospitalizations in facilities changed from prolonged stays (a timetable of years would not be unusual), to acute, shorter stays of 5-10 days.

Where do we go from here? It would be ideal to see well-built, safe, fully employed psychiatric hospitals popping up in needed communities around the country. In fact, there is research being conducted to help communities estimate how many beds they may need to shift the needle (Ryan K. McBain, Jonathan H. Cantor, & Nicole K. Eberhart, 2022).

But the obstacles to this are great, and it's probably not an attainable goal in the near future. A more manageable option would be placing greater priority on psychiatric prevention. This would mean fewer at-risk patients slipping into a critical state for which they would require a bed in the first place. But even this more moderate option presents major obstacles. It would mean shaking the practice of managed care loose from its leading role in this blockbuster drama, and that means serious financial backing and Washington D.C. support.

So, there's not enough beds. What does this mean for the ER physician I mentioned above?

No beds for a psychiatric patient mean a bed taken up for an extended period of time during which another patient cannot be seen in the emergency room.

A colleague shared an astounding number. In an ER he works in, a patient waited 108 hours for a psychiatric bed. That was 108 hours, over four days, that bed couldn't be occupied by another person in an emergency medical situation. What's more, that's 108 hours that patient could not attend individual or group therapy, which is often available on psychiatric units. They may have been seen by the hospital psychiatrist, but there's no guarantee. No coping skills are being shared in the ER for 108 hours.

So now the ER physician is frustrated, the patient is frustrated. Everybody is frustrated.

So until the country moves towards building more hospitals and insurance approves longer hospitalizations, how can the bed crisis improve in the short-term?

In several communities, unfortunately, the criteria for hospitalization have only become stricter. Traditionally, the criteria needed for psychiatric inpatient hospitalization consists of a patient demonstrating *imminent* danger to self or others, or an inability to care for self. It used to be that a suicidal patient was *always* admitted to a psychiatric hospital. But because of the lack of beds, an emphasis on the *imminent* part of "imminent danger" is taking precedence. *Imminent* implies the patient, in the near future, will cause harm to themselves or others. Usually this consists of either having a plan to cause harm, having a time or date to do so, or (most commonly) enacting a plan but aborting and seeking help. In other words, a person must have already tried causing harm to themselves or others or be at the very precipice of doing so; the days of showing up to a psych hospital and reporting suicidal ideation with placid self-possession have long passed. While voluntary admission exists, the availability of the bed may not.

Lower levels of care, such as IOPs (Intensive Outpatient Programs) and PHPs (Partial Hospitalization Programs) are popping up more and more around the country. As mentioned in Access to Care, these facilities are designed to help those who do not meet the *imminent* criteria for hospitalization, but still require a higher level of care than a regular outpatient psychiatry clinic.

Other tools are being created to help the bed crisis.

In 2020, the Ohio Department of Mental Health and Addiction Services unveiled their online bed registry, which in real time shows bed availability across the state. The project was funded in part by a federal grant from the Substance Abuse and Mental Health Services Administration (SAMHSA). This program is a fantastic jump forward for doctors who are looking for beds for their patients. But as a patient, don't expect to log in to a web site and make a reservation like you're booking a hotel room at

Disney World. The tool is for clinicians in the ER or mental health clinics to better target *potential* bed availability faster than they could manually faxing and calling *all* the psychiatric units in the area.

While efforts are being made at the back-end, I wonder about the front-end of this issue. What about preventing the need for an inpatient psychiatric bed?

Let's visit with one more patient. Please meet Michelle. Michelle is not a real patient, but rather an amalgamation.

Michelle is a 34-year-old woman who came from a community mental health center where she had been going for her care for several years. At the center, she had a psychiatrist, a therapist, and a case manager. The case manager kept tabs on Michelle, making sure she was picking up her medications and going to her psychiatrist and therapist appointments. She often touched base with Michelle throughout the week to see how she was doing. With all four working together (Michelle included) under this robust system, Michelle by all accounts was in good shape. This care essentially disappeared, however, when Michelle's insurance changed from state-funded Medicaid to private insurance. She did not meet the criteria for these services, and she had to change clinics.

Enter a private practice clinic. A clinic with a psychiatrist, therapists, but without access to a social worker or case manager for more complex cases. If the patient's insurance included these services, this was ideal, but not readily available to the clinic.

This limitation was mentioned to Michelle when she first came to the clinic. Based on her intake with the therapist, there were concerns her needs were greater than the services available.

Frustrated by losing her previous clinic and the efforts made to find this clinic, Michelle responded to the concerns. "Listen, finding a psychiatrist who takes my insurance took me forever. I waited for this appointment. I like you. I'm staying."

Over the next few years, the mental health team gave Michelle the best care possible. But without that social worker or case manager, it was a constant struggle. What ensued was moments of stability for Michelle, to be contrasted with many hospitalizations. She had a history of abuse of various substances, most notably opioids. She was sober, however, and received opioid replacement medication (suboxone) at another clinic (It may be worth mentioning, in order to paint the full picture, that Michelle did seek psychiatric care at that clinic, but she did not connect well with their psychiatrist. She went looking for a new psychiatrist and found a private practice but maintained her suboxone treatment at that facility.). On top of her addiction issues, Michelle was diagnosed with borderline personality disorder and struggled with feelings of abandonment, emotional regulation, and frequent suicidal thoughts.

I'd like to pause here just briefly. I recognize I have presented two cases of borderline personality disorder (BPD), which could cause some confusion about the condition, and might also beg the question of why I am not presenting other serious conditions, like schizophrenia. After all, borderline personality disorder has an estimated prevalence of 1.8% of the general population; bipolar disorder and schizophrenia have similar estimated prevalences of 2.8% and 1.1%, respectively (National Institute of Mental Health, 2023; Treatment Advocacy Center, 2022). But despite their roughly similar appearances among the population, it is borderline personality disorder which can make up to 20% of those hospitalized in psychiatric facilities. The nature of the condition, much like other serious mental illnesses, causes severe symptoms with catastrophic chaos in one's life. The disorder is marked by a poor self-image, severe emotional disability, dysfunctional relationships, and frequent suicidal behaviors. Thus, these two cases are being utilized to highlight elements in the mental health system.

Back to Michelle. Over the years of her care, Michelle was often hospitalized. There were stretches where her hospital visits were monthly occurrences. She would stabilize briefly on medication, but then her symptoms would reemerge. What is also noteworthy is that, as of now, the recommended treatment for those with borderline personality disorder is psychotherapy, the option with the most research behind it being dialectical behavioral therapy (DBT). Co-morbid depression, anxiety, insomnia, and PTSD symptoms, usually related to the kind of childhood trauma that is frequently seen in those with borderline personality disorder, can be treated with medications. But there are few medications geared towards improving emotional swings, negative self-image, and difficulty in relationships. Of course, more research is developing towards pharmacologic options.

On one occasion during an appointment, Michelle was growing increasingly frustrated with her treatment. She was upset that she seemed to improve on a medication, then worsen, usually due to an environment or relationship trigger that would incite an emotional collapse. She would become suicidal and be hospitalized. Her medications would usually be changed, she would discharge after 4-6 days, and return home feeling sick from the many medications necessary to control her emotional outbursts on the inpatient unit.

To try and break this cycle, a different approach was considered. Her medications were reviewed, including those that were making her feel like a zombie. But a pivotal question came from her therapist; what would she like without going to the hospital frequently? An attainable short-term goal was set; could she maintain stability for one month without requiring hospitalization, with scheduled and consistent work with her therapist?

Three months passed and Michelle had managed to avoid hospitalization. She was taking care of herself, going to therapy appointments consistently, and getting out of the house. What was also notable was how proud she was of herself. At age 34, she had spent years of her life bouncing from one psychiatric hospital to another, never really feeling better physically or mentally.

I wish this had a happy ending, but unfortunately Michelle's improvement did not last. Her insurance had changed to Medicare. She was not keeping appointments. Her therapist went back to the drawing board.

And what ensued was extremely frustrating.

Enter residential care.

For clarification, "residential care" in mental health means any long-term care facility, geared usually towards a certain diagnosis or group of diagnoses. For example, I'm sure you've seen those commercials for gorgeous rehabilitation centers where the iron gate opens to a curved drive lined with palm trees taking you to an estate of luxurious mansions for "your home away from home." You may not be surprised to learn this image is not always reality, but let's focus on the basics for now. Besides the common residential care focused on addiction treatment, there exists residential care for those with personality disorders, most frequently, BPD. But a roadblock exists here: Medicare does not cover residential care facilities. So while frequent hospitalizations will be covered, which was demonstrated in Michelle's history to not improve her overall health and resulted in continued need for acute care, the investment into a residential care stay, for 3-6 months or longer, to target Michelle's core issues with intensive therapy and medication management to reduce her risk of further hospitalization and improve her quality of life is not. Make this make sense.

We are talking about money. Money needs to be allocated for the current vacancy of long-term residential treatment options for those with serious mental health issues.

I propose a multi-level model comprised of long-term inpatient hospitalization (greater than 1 year), midterm inpatient hospitalization (greater than 3 months) and acute care hospitalization (less than 1 month). An augmentation of this plan could be the inclusion of group homes. But as we see from

Geraldo's work and the *New York Times* follow-up article, it is not just about the facility. It is about the care given. This is where the money comes in as well. In Geraldo's footage of Willowbrook he commented there was one staff member for many patients. While I acknowledge staffing and good care is a plight that all care facilities, mental health or not, are battling, I am encouraging that the safety, treatment, and wellbeing of those with mental health, and those who care for these patients, is addressed at the highest priority. The ripples of this endeavor can improve many avenues of our society and *it* is the humane thing to do.

So imagine: a metal scale, with two metal plates on each side, awaiting an object to weigh against the other. On one side, prevention, where Michelle can go to a residential care facility for 3, 6, 9 or maybe 12 months to receive extensive psychotherapy targeting elements of her personality and psyche, while also helping her learn coping skills she never learned as a child or a young adult. On the other side of the scale lies Michelle's current treatment, an existence of expensive and frequent hospitalizations, sometimes even ER visits, with exhausting medication changes and prescriptions, clinic visits, and therapy visits. Which side should we choose? I would wager that money spent on Michelle's frequent hospital visits on investments in Michelle's mental health from a preventative nature. It's my professional opinion this would result not only in an improved and possibly productive Michelle, but even a lower cost--which is what matters to the insurance industry. So when will the insurance companies use their manpower to analyze these options, instead of stamping refusals and denials on treatment that is going nowhere? I don't have the answer, but as the clinician invested in Michelle's wellbeing, her future is at risk, and the scale needs to shift.

American Psychiatric Association (Producer). (2022, May). "The Psychiatric Bed Crisis in the US: Understanding the Problem and Moving Toward Solutions". Retrieved from https://www.psychiatry.org/getmedia/81f685f1-036e-4311-8dfc-e13ac425380f/APA-Psychiatric-Bed-Crisis-Report-Full.pdf

Autism Speaks (Producer). (2020, March 26). CDC estimate on autism prevalence increases by nearly 10 percent, to 1 in 54 children in the U.S. Retrieved from https://www.autismspeaks.org/press-release/cdc-estimate-autism-prevalence-increases-nearly-10-percent-1-54-children-us

Disability Justice. (2022). The Closing of Willowbrook. In.

National Institute of Mental Health (Producer). (2023). "Bipolar Disorder". Retrieved from https://www.nimh.nih.gov/health/statistics/bipolar-disorder

Rivera, G. (Writer). (1972). Willowbrook: The Last Great Disgrace. In. WABC-TV Channel 7.

Ryan K. McBain, P., MPH1, Jonathan H. Cantor, P., & Nicole K. Eberhart, P. (Producer). (2022, February 16). "Estimating Psychiatric Bed Shortages in the US". Retrieved from https://jamanetwork.com/journals/jamapsychiatry/fullarticle/2789297#:~:text=The%20US%20has%2021%20psychiatric,respect%20to%20psychiatric%20bed%20numbers

Torrey, E., & Zdanowicz, M. (2014, April 8). The treatment of persons with mental illness in prisons and jails: A state survey.

Treatment Advocacy Center (Producer). (2022). "Schizophrenia - Fact Sheet". Retrieved from https://www.treatmentadvocacycenter.org/evidence-and-research/learn-more-about/25-schizophrenia-fact-sheet#:~:text=Although%20it%20affects%20barely%201,States%20aged%2018%20or%20older.

Weiser, B. (Producer). (2020, February 21). "Beatings, Burns and Betrayal: The Willowbrook Scandal's Legacy". *The New York Times.* Retrieved from https://www.nytimes.com/2020/02/21/nyregion/willowbrook-state-school-staten-island.html

Zeliadt, N. (Producer). (2019). Children with severe autism increasingly overlooked in research. *Spectrum News.* Retrieved from https://www.spectrumnews.org/news/children-severe-autism-increasingly-overlooked-research/

This Isn't Working

Chapter Four

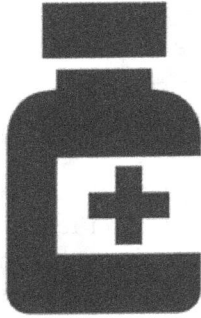

Xannies

"What time is it?", Kinley asked me, during a one-hour initial evaluation which was now going past 90 minutes.

"It's 12:20pm," I answered.

"Oh, I'm late for my dose!" she said, referring to her alprazolam (Xanax) prescription.

Kinley was a petite 73-year-old woman, wearing leather pants, a bright pink sweater, and smelling slightly of cigarette smoke.

Twenty-six years ago, Kinley's OB-GYN physician had prescribed her a drug called alprazolam, popularly known as Xanax, for anxiety she experienced after the loss of her mother.

She explained to me that she initially only took it as needed, but soon found the doses she was taking were not as effective. Kinley's OG-GYN increased her dose, and increased it again, until she was taking scheduled doses 5 times a day.

Hence why, at 12:20pm, she was concerned about the time.

I asked Kinley how she was feeling that moment. "I'm feeling nervous. I don't feel okay." I explained to Kinley that she was likely experiencing a minor withdrawal due to being late with her dose. She asked to know more.

According to several studies, there are two natural chemicals in her brain responsible for how she was feeling: GABA and glutamate.

The way I explain these chemicals to my patients is this: GABA is a calming chemical in our brain and body. When GABA receptors (there are many with different effects), but to keep this simple, are active, calming effect is achieved. Alcohol and benzodiazepines both act on the GABA receptors, both eliciting a calming effect (also slow down commands, such as take less breaths). When the GABA receptors are not being targeted, as in alcohol withdrawal, or benzodiazepine withdrawal, this leaves glutamate, the excitatory chemical that is GABA's opposite, still active. The glutamate is thought to be partially responsible for the symptoms of withdrawal (uneasiness, anxiety, restlessness, and in severe situations, the possibility of death, usually by arrhythmia) (Tsuda, Shimizu, & Suzuki, 1999).

Kinley looked at me a little bewildered. In fact, at first, I thought she looked a bit upset.

"So you're telling me that I am experiencing anxiety because I'm late on the medication that is supposed to help with anxiety?" Kinley asked.

"Yes, that is what I am saying." (This is a conversation I have multiple times a week).

Kinley was sizing me up. She was already on a regimen of Lexapro (escitalopram) on top of the alprazolam. Further medication was unlikely to help with her anxiety, but detoxing might. I convinced her to let me help her taper off from the alprazolam, which is no easy feat. It's a process that can take several months, and in some situations, a year or more. But I had seen good success with several other patients, and they had been relieved to free themselves of reliance on alprazolam.

After 90 minutes of discussion, she said, "I trust you. Let's do this."

First, a quick medical minute: what exactly *is* alprazolam? Alprazolam belongs to a family of medications called *benzodiazepines*. They primarily boost neuroreceptors for the neurotransmitter 'GABA,' which is a calming chemical.

There are many benzodiazepines, but some common and recognizable iterations are diazepam, lorazepam, clonazepam, and temazepam. You may know these as Valium, Ativan, Klonopin, and Restoril, respectively.

The benzodiazepine alprazolam, brand name Xanax, was approved in 1981 by the FDA (Food and

Drug Administration) for use in patients with anxiety and panic disorder.

Its purpose was, and is, to act like a rescue medication. like an inhaler works for one with asthma. Xanax is intended to rescue patients with panic attacks. Consider: A panic attack is setting in, and the patient is not able to function normally. They may be experiencing shortness of breath, chest pain, increased heart rate, and, according to the criteria for panic attack diagnosis, the feeling of impending doom--as if they feel they may die.

The idea is the patient would take alprazolam to abort this attack and restore ability to function. Those who have panic disorder, whose criteria include frequent and debilitating panic attacks, could use alprazolam to function normally.

What subsequently happened was the beginnings of overprescribing of the medication. Alprazolam was never intended to become the general treatment for anxiety, although its original intent for use included general anxiety. But as general anxiety was listed as a reason to prescribe alprazolam, that (perhaps unsurprisingly) became the norm. Alprazolam was prescribed for anyone and everyone who had anxiety. And so, by the 1970s, even before its FDA approval for the purpose of anxiety, alprazolam had become widely abused (H. Ashton, 2005).

The American Psychiatric Associated finally recognized benzodiazepine dependence as a diagnosis in 1990 (C. Salzman, 1991). This problem continues today. In 2004, in the United States alone, there were 17.9 million prescriptions for alprazolam. This rose to a high of 28.9 million prescriptions in 2014 (Mikulic,

2022). In 2014, there were 317 million people in the United States. (Schlesinger, 2013). This means that, statistically, in 2014, 1 in every 10 Americans was given a prescription for alprazolam!

Overuse of alprazolam carries major risks. Alprazolam, as discussed, by way of multiple neurochemical reactions, increases GABA uptake, the calming chemical in the brain. This affects more than just mood. GABA works on parts of the brain that control unconscious bodily functions such as breathing. What can result with overuse is, to put it simply, an overabundance of GABA that floods the brain telling critical areas, "Hey! Cool down, we don't need you to work so hard." That's all fine when someone is experiencing a panic attack, and the brain is telling the lungs and heart to slow down so a person can breathe normally and have a normal heart rate. But with overuse, over time the lungs can essentially lose the message to breathe, also known as respiratory depression.

This is not theoretical; respiratory depression is a major cause of death in substance overdose. A hot topic currently is opioids. The opioid crisis. Opioids cause a similar issue with overuse, by sending messages from the brain to the lungs by way of different chemical messengers. What statistics and widespread prescribing of benzodiazepines is telling us is this: prepare for the benzodiazepine crisis.

There is a general consensus in the medical community that, while opioids are currently the foremost concern for the increase in deaths related to pain medication overuse, benzodiazepines are soon to follow as a recognized risk for death. This is not to say there is not already concern; there is. Currently, 49 states have implemented prescription drug monitoring programs (PDMP) to prevent patients or drug abusers from stockpiling, "doctor-shopping", overusing controlled medications, including benzodiazepines (Holmgren, Botelho, & Brandt, 2020).

It's worth it to talk about PDMPs in more detail. To do that, let's consider Tom.

Tom is a (hypothetical) 49-year-old male who is seen in the emergency room for a broken arm. He is about to be discharged with 12 pills of an opioid. This prescription is intended for Tom to take every 4-6 hours for severe pain until he can be seen by the orthopedic surgeon in clinic. Prior to this prescription being sent to the pharmacy, however, the prescribing physician must check the PDMP's online portal to check Tom's currently prescribed controlled medications. Red flags could be that Tom already is on pain medications that he did not disclose to the ER and has filled 120 tablets of an opioid 3 weeks ago and should have enough at home to help with his ailment. Others include "doctor shopping" which could look like multiple physicians writing frequent prescriptions for opioids. Current national guidelines, including those by CMS and FDA, recommend that co-prescribing benzodiazepines and opioids are limited in most situations. And in those situations that require both, physicians are advised to institute close monitoring to forestall overuse.

The PDMP is one of the most useful tools to come out of the digital age of medicine. The ability to understand a patient's controlled medication history can help thwart unnecessary prescribing, check compliance with current prescriptions, and (and I feel this most affects how I practice) allow a treating team to know what medications a patient is taking when they show up in the ER unresponsive or, often in cases of the elderly, confused with no medical information. Finding that the patient is on one or more controlled substances prior to arrival to the hospital can help with diagnosis, or also prevent a dangerous withdrawal.

So we mentioned overuse as a major risk of benzodiazepines like alprazolam.

Another is withdrawal. I will never forget this one case from my residency. I was on call and called to the hospital floor for an urgent consult. A 48-year-old man had been admitted to the hospital with confusion. He was becoming increasingly confused and was hallucinating. The work-up thus far, including labs and brain imaging, was unremarkable.

On checking with the family, the primary team had learned that the patient is prescribed diazepam (valium), a benzodiazepine, outside the hospital. There was concern he could be withdrawing.

Upon my arrival to the hospital floor, I recall checking my paper to see what room the gentleman was in. But I actually could hear my patient before I ever reached his room. The sound of what sounded like a dog barking was reverberating down the hallway. At first, I thought this might be a therapy dog. But while therapy dogs are often on the hospital floor for patient comfort, they are invariably extremely well-trained. I have never heard one bark.

As I walked down the hallway, the barking was increasingly louder. I had found the room I was supposed to go to. I entered the room and found a middle-aged gentleman…barking. When asked what was happening, he stated he was trying to get his dog, Rufus, to answer him. After many minutes of de-escalating the patient, I found two bits of important information. First, I found that he was taking more diazepam than his doctor was prescribing. And second, I found he had not had any diazepam at all in 3 days.

His delirious state was a direct result of benzodiazepine withdrawal.

Substance withdrawal from benzodiazepines is as dangerous as alcohol withdrawal for a heavy alcoholic. Initially, patients can become anxious, like Kinley, with some heart racing (tachycardia), and most often, tremor. You hear about the "shakes" sometimes on movies or TV. These are usually upper extremity tremors, sometimes lower extremity, that start 12-18 hours after a person who consistently uses alcohol has stopped drinking. For benzodiazepines, the window is usually longer; sometimes it takes up to 5 days from the last dose before withdrawal symptoms can start.

As the time goes on between last use of alcohol or benzodiazepines, the withdrawal symptoms can become more severe. Confusion can set in. Blood pressure can rise. Heart rate can increase. Hallucinations are frequent. Risk of seizure increases. Death can even result from a seizure that does not stop, or more frequently a heart arrhythmia.

So, when a patient is prescribed a high dose of daily benzodiazepines for "anxiety", it can be understood why there is concern about the overprescribing of these medications.

I think the most natural question could be in the context of 2024, how was all this impacted by the COVID-19 pandemic?

Initially, studies seemed to show that prescriptions of benzodiazepines were on the decrease. Reasons for this include a temporary decrease in elective surgeries at the first of the pandemic. Benzodiazepines are sometimes prescribed for anxiety and nausea related to surgery. Others cite a gap in mental health care as the world adjusted to more virtual care with the pandemic. Yet as the pandemic has continued, studies have shown a worrying increase in the number of benzodiazepine prescriptions. But as with the opioid problem, the monitoring of prescriptions, especially by state and federal drug agencies, is also increasing. Physicians and mid-level practitioners (APRN, PA) are receiving more oversight for the number of controlled substance prescriptions.

So how do I prescribe benzodiazepines?

With great caution.

I see patients in my practice with multiple medical conditions, and often with cancer. Oftentimes these conditions call for pain medications.

First, I treat anxiety according to the guidelines of anxiety treatment. Antidepressants (something of a misnomer, I explain frequently to my patients) is actually a treatment for anxiety. Often times, therapy is highly encouraged, especially for those with other anxiety conditions like phobias or social anxiety. While a majority of patients will respond to an antidepressant--noticing they feel less worried, irritable, restless--sometimes they do not. New research is looking at psychiatric medications from other categories that can be used to help anxiety. With patients who describe panic attacks, I do prescribe benzodiazepines, as they are in the guidelines of treatment for panic attacks and panic disorder. But the number is often limited and comes with close monitoring. In psychiatry, there is a fine balance between treating the symptoms the patient reports, but also encouraging the patient, through psychotherapy, to use the mind in a way to help manage the anxiety they feel.

We, as a society, are anxious. We are overstimulated, overspent, chemical'ed up. Looking at you, coffee-drinkers at 4pm. Our evolving brains were not ready to be pelleted with news, social media, the expectation of 24/7 availability, complex modern financial constraints, and to top it off, an international pandemic one would see in the movies.

We are, psychologically, becoming Swiss-cheesed.

My father, a medical doctor who self-describes as a student of psychiatry, has 45+ years of clinical practice seeing thousands of patients over those years. He came home one day and said we are all donkeys, and we are carrying too much. He then showed me a picture he found on a google search.

A man is sitting in a buggy, with cartons upon cartons behind him. The donkey is in front, but instead of all four legs secured planted on the ground, they are in the air, forced by the weight of the buggy. He turned to me, furrowing his brow, and said, "Stop being the donkey. Lighten up your load."

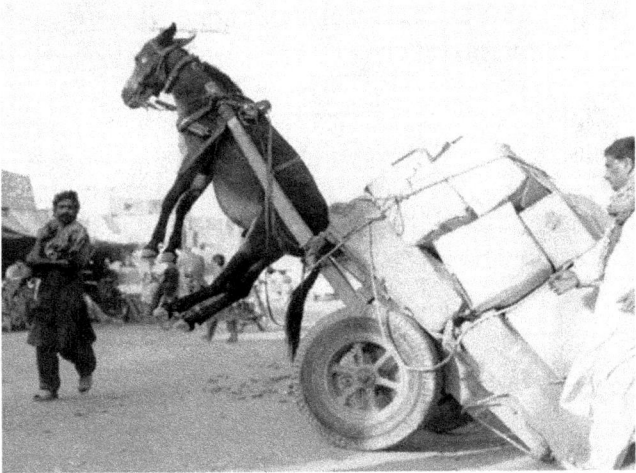

(Ranchers.net, 2004)

There is a new danger that emerges when anxiety becomes so commonplace. Anxiety is becoming stereotyped. Timeworn. This is not to discount the struggle anxiety brings, but when our shared cultural concept of anxiety devolves into a simplistic stereotype, we demand simplistic solutions. In truth, identifying the emotion is only the first part.

So, what am I trying to bring home with this chapter?

Should alprazolam be banned? No. Medicating can help anxiety and is a useful tool in combatting panic attacks. But are we going to see benzodiazepines become a focus for overuse prevention in the near future? Yes. If you are taking alprazolam does this mean you need to go throw it away? No, please again read the risk of withdrawal.

But as a psychiatrist who does spend a majority of work finding the right medication regimen for my patients, I am saying, we need to do more than just turn to a pill. Because a pill, after all, cannot always solve the problem.

Let's close out this chapter by closing out Kinley's story. After 9 months of frequent visits and reassurance, Kinley sauntered in for a visit wearing a fluffy fur coat, bright pink lipstick, with a grin I had not seen before. I knew why she was grinning.

"Doctor, we did it!" Kinley exclaimed.

After 26 years and 9 months or so of daily alprazolam use, Kinley was off alprazolam.

I shared with Kinley my observations of patients similar to her, unknowingly physically addicted to a medication that was intended to help but wasn't. I commented that I hoped to write an article about cases like hers. She quickly signed off on her case being used, but with one caveat.

She said, "Call me Kinley. I've always loved that name."

C. Salzman. (1991). The APA Task Force report on benzodiazepine dependence, toxicity, and abuse. *Am J Psychiatry*, 148:151-152.

H. Ashton. (2005). The diagnosis and management of benzodiazepine dependence. *Curr Opin Psychiatry*, 18:249-255.

Holmgren, A. J., Botelho, A., & Brandt, A. M. (2020). A history of prescription drug monitoring programs in the United States: Political appeal and public health efficacy. *American journal of public health, 110*(8), 1191-1197.

Mikulic, M. (Producer). (2022, February 4). Number of alprazolam prescriptions in the U.S. from 2004 to 2019 (in millions) *Statista*. Retrieved from https://www.statista.com/statistics/781816/alprazolam-sodium-prescriptions-number-in-the-us/

Ranchers.net (Producer). (2004, 11-6-2023). Overworked Donkey. Retrieved from https://www.ranchers.net/jokes/overworked.htm

Schlesinger, R. (Producer). (2013, December 31). The 2014 U.S. and World Populations. *US News*. Retrieved from https://www.usnews.com/opinion/blogs/robert-schlesinger/2013/12/31/us-population-2014-317-million-and-71-billion-in-the-world

Tsuda, M., Shimizu, N., & Suzuki, T. (1999). Contribution of glutamate receptors to benzodiazepine withdrawal signs. *The Japanese Journal of Pharmacology, 81*(1), 1-6.

This Isn't Working

Chapter Five

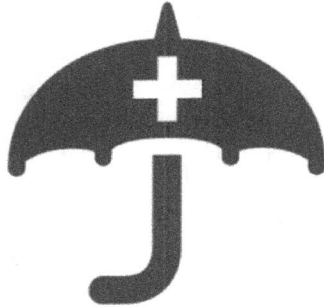

Who You Gonna Call?!

I often encounter the same memes around March. The younger generation attests that they didn't need trigonometry in school, they needed tax classes! Well, here's another class that may be needed: End of life planning.

I'd like to tell you a story about a patient named Greg. Details have been adjusted.

Greg was a 69-year-old man, with near blindness, admitted to our academic hospital from an outside facility because the sodium level in his blood was too high. This was causing a change in his mental status. He was intermittently confused, aka delirious.

On Day 23 of his hospitalization, the psychiatry consult and liaison team, including yours truly, was contacted for a consult.

The case manager who was trying to find him a facility to discharge to, as Greg was now medically stable, and needed to know the patient's ability to pay for the facility. You just don't get to discharge somewhere for free from a hospital.

Before we proceed, we're going to run into some terminology here in this chapter. And if you're wondering why this is different from the Geraldo Rivera chapter story, just hear me out.

So, Greg was refusing to sign a document that allows the case manager to talk to Greg's bank. You see, she needed to assess his financial abilities to pay for a nursing home.

Fun game here: do you know who will pay for your nursing home care? If you don't have Medicaid, it will be *you*. Though Medicaid covers 100% of nursing home costs, the program is strictly means-tested. Most estimates put the percentage of nursing home costs currently being covered by Medicaid at between 45 and 65% (Paying for Senior Care, 2021).

If you're hoping Medicare may pick up the slack, think again. Medicare will pay for short-term care, sometimes called skilled nursing facilities, for a time long enough to recover from an acute illness. According to Medicaid, that takes about 30 days; after that, the patient is responsible for a portion of the daily cost of the stay("Paying for Nursing Home Care: Medicare, Medicaid & Other Assistance," 2021).

Now that we have a better grasp of what was facing our friend Greg, let's get back to his case.

Greg had been fluctuating in his willingness to release his financial records to his case worker. Speaking to the attending physician on morning rounds, Greg had agreed to sign any relevant papers needed so the case manager could speak to his bank. By afternoon, Greg had become aggressive and was refusing to cooperate. Hence, there was concern he was not understanding the situation completely. So, a capacity consult was requested. It's not unusual for decision-making capacity evaluations to be a part of discharge planning. For instance, a patient may demand they be discharged when their condition is too severe for them to live independently at home with no supportive care.

Key Definition: *capacity evaluation*

Psychiatrists are usually consulted in the hospital for a "capacity evaluation." The full description is the psychiatrist performs an evaluation to assess if a patient can make certain medical decisions. For example, a patient with cancer is confused in the hospital from a medical issue, aka delirious. He is needing to receive chemotherapy in the hospital for his cancer, but suddenly, refuses. His oncologist, who knows the patient well, is surprised by this, as the patient had been very clear with his intent to continue chemotherapy for a diagnosis that has a good prognosis. The psychiatrist is then notified of the situation. The purpose of the evaluation is to assess if the patient can understand his current medical condition, the proposed recommendations, the risks/benefits of this recommendation and whether the patient has a clear choice regarding this decision. Ultimately, it is also assessed if any outlying factors could be affecting the patient's decision-making capacity, such as delirium, depression. The key to these assessments, which I must remind others of frequently, is that this is a very concise evaluation for a very specific question. These assessments have no resemblance to a person's competency. Competency, often a term encountered in the judicial system, is an understanding of a patient's full capacity to essentially make any decisions for themselves. Competency is determined in the courtroom by a judge, not a psychiatrist in the hospital.

We assessed Greg. Initially, he did demonstrate some confusion. He had trouble describing the treatment he had received thus far, or even explaining why he was in the hospital to begin with. Once he was informed, he demonstrated the ability to grasp and manipulate this information back to us when he was asked again. This showed some retention of information. He was very cooperative, even kind, and said he was happy to work with the case manager. At the time of the assessment, although he had previously had some fluctuations in his cooperativeness, he was demonstrating ability to participate in discharge planning. Of course, this evaluation happened a bit later in the day, after the case manager had left. So what do you think happened the next day?

When the case manager returned the next morning with the paperwork, Greg went level 10. He was again completely uncooperative. We returned for another assessment. The Greg we found was very different from the Greg we'd had a pleasant conversation with the previous day. He was confused and agitated. He did not want to work with the case worker; what he wanted was a popsicle. Once we had delivered a strawberry popsicle, we reassessed him. He was not grasping information and could not state a clear choice about what the options were for discharge.

At this point, also because of his fluctuating capacity, we deemed that at this time, he did not demonstrate decision-making capacity to participate in discharge planning.

So if the patient cannot decide for themselves, who decides for them?

This depends on what state you are in for the details, but broadly speaking, the surrogate decision maker will usually be the next of kin. This part is important: this is in the situation that the patient does not already have a health care power of attorney or court-appointed guardian document in place.

Let's talk next of kin. Again, the rules of order on who is next of kin depends on the state, but usually they are the patient's spouse or domestic partner, then their adult child, parent, sibling, and so on. Some states do have room for a close friend to be next of kin.

So consider: if someone's only family is a sister with whom they've have zero contact after some huge falling out 20 years ago, and they land in the hospital after a motor vehicle accident with a head injury with resulting confusion, and a non-emergent issue arises that it is felt a family member should be considered to help decide, this sister could be the next of kin to make that decision. For Greg, this was exactly the case.

One could understand the importance of this key factor in one's health care. It isn't just about having health insurance, a primary care clinician, or a pharmacy you like, it's also planning for when things are not going well in other areas; who is going to make decisions for you, if you cannot?

Greg's sister was contacted as his next of kin. Happily, she was prepared to set the past aside to provide the help her brother needed. But that proved to be the last of the easy hurdles. We had hoped to have Greg discharged that afternoon. What ensued for the *thirty days* Greg was in the hospital, medically stable and clinically ready for discharge, was a never-ending back and forth between the case manager and Greg's sister on pursuing guardianship. The bank needed documents stating the sister could access the patient's bank accounts. So, she is given a detailed document of forty-three pages to start filling out, and quickly. Because if you've lost count, Greg had been in the hospital at this point for more than 50 days. And because his behavior had been fluctuating, and at times he had even been physically aggressive with the nursing staff, he had been confined to his room. Hospitals ensure that all patients are treated humanely and with respect. It is taken very seriously. But this poor gentleman is stuck. Spending one night in the hospital is bad enough. Imagine being there for almost two months. Not because you're healing or being treated, but because of legalities. And the visit hadn't been free up until then, either. The cost of this stay was piling up.

At this point, Greg's case manager was dealing with pressure from both the hospital and his insurance to get him discharged. Greg's sister was fumbling tirelessly through the guardianship papers. And all we had managed to do for Greg was to switch him to sugar-free popsicles to keep his blood sugar from spiking from all his popsicle consumption.

The court was contacted, and the judge allowed a pivot to expedite the discharge efforts. A physician can officially document the need for the sister to have guardianship of Greg. So as the consulting psychiatrist, we were brought in to do another assessment. But this one is different. It was time to assess the patient past the *specific* decision-making capacity. The patient's *full* decision-making capacity was being considered. As in, his ability to make *any* decisions.

Now you may be frightened to know this is possible, and indeed, the situation is ripe for abuse. If you have seen the movie on Netflix "I Care a Lot", you know the worst-case scenario. Spoiler alert for those who have missed the movie; the main character, played extremely well by actress Rosamund Pike, has a company where she serves as a court appointed guardian. Her network of physicians and the trust by the court leads her to hand-selecting "cherries", who are wealthy women with no family who now need a guardian. As you can imagine, with her court appointed powers, she essentially robs these women. Trouble ensues, Peter Dinklage shows up, and the story becomes unbelievable, but the point is, this is obviously serious. By the way, Rosamund Pike's character gets what she deserves... (Blakeson, 2020)

A letter was created supporting the need for a guardian for this patient and submitted to the court, like the movie. But in this case, it is the patient's sister who is going to make the decisions for the patient.

But if the sister did not exist, a court-appointed guardian (i.e., a Rosamund Pike) would be the next option.

So how could this entire debacle have been avoided?

By a few silly sheets of paper.

If Greg had ever been given the opportunity to fill out a healthcare power of attorney document, or health care proxy, this document would have come into effect when Greg was not able to make his own medical decisions. If he had not wanted his sister or next of kin to be in that role, the healthcare power of attorney could specify for him who would be.

It's worth noting that a power of attorney document could empower his preferred agent in financial decisions related to his care as well.

So essentially, if Greg had been in possession of a power of attorney document that had been created at a time when he was mentally sound, this kerfuffle could have been avoided.

As the title of the chapter asks, *"Who you gonna call?"*

Reader, have you heard of a power of attorney?

Do you need a lawyer for this? Not technically. It is suggested that one may seek counsel for advice regarding the paperwork, but a lawyer is not necessary to fill out the paperwork.

Once you have this document, if you are ever admitted to the hospital, you may be asked if you have a power of attorney. Would be good to say you do. Also, some carry in their wallet a card that states who the power of attorney is in the event you are unconscious on arrival to the hospital.

Let's move on with Greg's story.

Nursing homes. Dementia. The future.

Greg, after continued clinical evaluation, was determined to have a neurocognitive disorder (aka dementia). I will not even act like I can do justice to the 122 page "Alzheimer's Disease Facts and Figures" report that can be found on the Alzheimer's Association website. This report so perfectly targets all areas that those of us in healthcare are worried about: the prevalence, the caregivers, the workforce and the health care costs.

By 2050, the number of people age 65 and older with Alzheimer's dementia is projected to reach 12.7 million.

Projected Number of People Age 65 and Older (Total and by Age) in the U.S. Population with Alzheimer's Dementia, 2020 to 2060

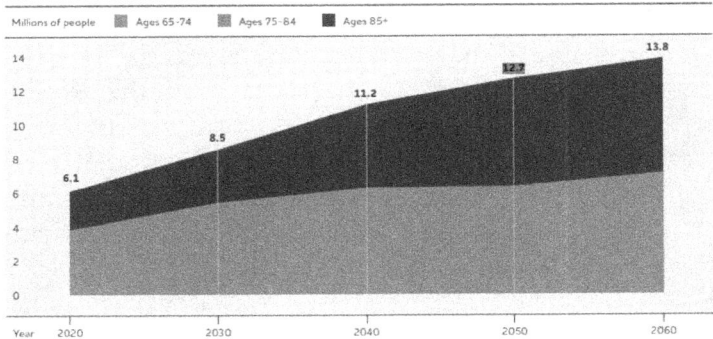

(Alzheimer's Association, 2023)

While living in a country of 331 million people, 12.7 million may not sound daunting, but if you consider the ripples of a diagnosis of Alzheimer's dementia, like cost, the situation becomes grimmer. The total lifetime cost of care for someone with dementia was estimated at $377,621 in 2021 dollars. Seventy percent of the lifetime cost of care is borne by family caregivers in the forms of unpaid caregiving and out-of-pocket expenses for items ranging from medications to food for the person with dementia.

In 2022, the total national cost of caring for people living with Alzheimer's and other dementias is projected to reach $321 billion.*

*Does not include the $271.6 billion in unpaid caregiving by family and friends.

What can we expect for 2050?

Just under $1 trillion in 2050 (in 2022 dollars).

In today's climate where the national debt seems like a cartoon, in which the main character is sitting at the accountant's desk, typing zero after zero on a calculator, as the other cartoon character's jaw drops as the paper swirls on the desk then fills the office to the brim, leaving the characters gasping for air, 1 trillion seems like a problem. Especially when you remind yourself, we are talking about one diagnosis, for one demographic of the society...cue the shocked eye wide open emoji.

For the sake of brevity, I will just say we should be worried. Alzheimer's, while the most common type of dementia, does not even account for all neurocognitive disorders. Tack on studies recently released regarding COVID-19 and subsequent brain health, we are looking at a severe health care crisis.

In American culture, at least, the concept of the elderly "staying at home with family" has fallen out of favor. Space is tight. Finances are limited. Some simply cannot imagine taking on that role while working and caring for their immediate family. The concept of the "village" has changed with families strewn across a connected country and world. Families often no longer live in close proximity. So in the modern world, what options are available as our population gets older and independent living becomes impossible?

I mentioned this earlier regarding those with serious mental illness, or those with severe autism or other intellectual disabilities, who could not live independently. But now we are including another group who needs help in that area: Those with dementia.

Group homes can serve, to an extent. But as the brain progressively declines, any element of independence must be limited. Nursing homes, memory care centers, whatever you want to call them, will be needed in greater numbers than they currently exist.

Fun facts about geriatric psychiatric facilities. These are psychiatric inpatient units specifically for those usually age 65+, with a neurocognitive disorder. But the caveat is, as explained earlier about inpatient psychiatric units, these are not total care facilities. As of now, criteria for gero-psych units require a patient to be able to both ambulate (that's doctor-speak for walking independently or with minor assistance, such as with a cane or walker), and be able to complete what we call ADL/IADL. This stands for "activities of daily living" and "independent activities of daily living." Think getting dressed, using the toilet, eating. Of course, for patients with advanced dementia, both ambulation and ADL/IADL are both out of reach.

You can understand that this limits admission to a small group of those with dementia.

I should explain why someone is admitted to a gero-psych unit. Oftentimes, it is for behavioral issues related to dementia. Agitation, hallucinations, elopement (see leaving the home or hospital when they're not supposed to, NOT getting married in Vegas!), etc. Here's a super-quick example: Mary has dementia and lives with her daughter, and she is leaving the house at night. On one night, Mary became extremely agitated when she was being guided home. Mary would be admitted to a gero-psych unit for short-term medication adjustments so she can safely return to living with daughter for the time being.

Also, those who are 65+ with a psychiatric diagnosis (schizophrenia, bipolar disorder) can be treated at these facilities.

What should be considered moving forward?

In the patients I encounter with dementia with behavioral issues, it is my job, as a psychiatrist, to target the behavioral issues. Treating the dementia itself falls under the purview of the neurologist. I help dementia patients sleep, cease hallucinating, be less aggressive, and ultimately allow them to potentially stay home longer.

I have come across situations where I felt the care was as ideal as possible. Neurologist referred patient to me. Patient was seeing neurologist and psychiatrist (me) frequently. Patient's mental status declined. Home health initiated so nursing came to the house for several hours a day to help the patient and give the caregiver some reprieve. Patient declined further. Home hospice initiated. Patient passed peacefully at home.

This gently sloping transition, however, does not represent the majority of cases. For one thing, don't assume the family will have the financial or time resources to care for the patient at home.

I remember encountering a family in the hospital facing such life-changing decisions regarding their mother, Helen. Helen's functioning was declining due to dementia, and her family was not able to care for her at home. The case manager, hospice nurse, and physician were working with them and the patient to find the ideal place for the patient to go. But Helen's family had limited funds. Helen did not have significant savings, and she had not filled out Medicaid paperwork that had been suggested to her by her family physician several years ago. So while the case manager was fervently helping the family fill out the Medicaid paperwork, the patient needed somewhere to go. They were given a list of nursing homes to consider. Luckily, in some situations, the nursing homes will accept a patient knowing Medicaid will be accepted and can help pay for some of the stay even prior to the approval.

I remember hearing about a ranking system for these nursing homes. CMS gives a certain number of "stars" to care centers, based on their survey and reports (CMS.gov, 2022). As one would expect, the higher-rated nursing homes were more costly. Of course, any family would want their family member to be at the "5 star" nursing home, but when faced with potential costs, may end up with a 2- or 3-star facility. Imagine knowing you can only afford to place your mother in a facility that may have a history of violations or safety concerns?

I think there are a couple of things to suggest here.

Number 1, if this is all news to you and you thought your health insurance or Medicare that you pay into every year was going to pay for your Florida nursing home, where oranges grow on trees outside and the crashing of waves puts you to sleep at night, please read further.

Moving away from the financial aspects--where are all these patients with dementia going to go? Gero-psych units and nursing homes may need to join forces.

Med-psych (medicine-psychiatric) units are slowly popping up. These units, while considered safe, have more abilities to treat those with medical conditions that may prohibit placement into a psychiatric facility.

So somehow combining the expertise of geriatricians, geriatric psychiatrists, physical therapists, occupational therapists, speech therapists, counselors all into one facility could better address the needs and provide continuity. Then, attached inpatient hospice in comfortable settings where family could potentially stay with the patient could further build on this synergy. But this operation would be difficult, not just logistically, but financially.

Again, what have we learned is the bottom line with these proposals? Money. How will we get it? Here's one suggestion to get the ball rolling: allocations from taxes and Medicare withholdings should have a separate payment plan where you pay into future mental health services. And if you don't end up needing these mental health services, they roll into your Medicare available funds for general health. We need to start realizing that blanket funds for "health care" are not going to address the large costs that make up so much of our overall health care costs.

Alzheimer's Association (Producer). (2023). Alzheimer's Disease Facts and Figures. Retrieved from https://www.alz.org/media/Documents/alzheimers-facts-and-figures.pdf

Blakeson, J. (Writer). (2020). I Care a Lot. In: Netflix.

CMS.gov. (2022). Five-Star Quality Rating System. Retrieved from https://www.cms.gov/medicare/health-safety-standards/certification-compliance/five-star-quality-rating-system

Paying for Nursing Home Care: Medicare, Medicaid & Other Assistance. (2021, June 16). *Paying for Senior Care*. Retrieved from https://www.payingforseniorcare.com/nursing-homes

Paying for Senior Care. (2021, June 16). Paying for Nursing Home Care: Medicare, Medicaid & Other Assistance. Retrieved from https://www.payingforseniorcare.com/nursing-homes

This Isn't Working

101

Chapter Six

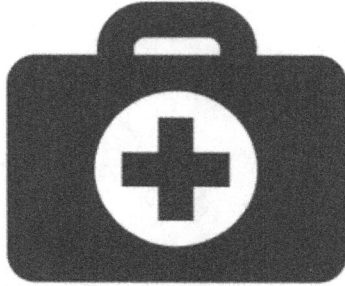

The Aid to Medicaid

"Do you see patients with Medicaid?"

The receptionist answers this question multiple times a day. Those answering the phones at any private or hospital-funded mental health clinic in America will be familiar with this question. A quick look at some general data will illustrate why.

In October of 2020, the American Psychological Association reported on a tsunami wave of mental health issues linked to the stress of the COVID-19 pandemic. At the time, the APA warned of "a national mental health crisis that could yield serious health and social consequences for years to come."(American Psychological Association, 2020). In another report only a few months later, it described this wave of mental health problems as a "second pandemic," which was causing physical issues as well as mental ones. (American Psychological Association, 2021) Their findings were echoed by the Kaiser Family Foundation, who released a report at about the same time that adults with symptoms of anxiety and depression in January 2021 had quadrupled from where they were in early 2019 (Nirmita Panchal, 2021),

This "second pandemic" had measurable effects on the economy. Prior to the pandemic, a 2015 study found that major depressive disorder alone cost the economy $210.5 *billion*, with fully half of that attributed to a loss of workplace productivity. (Paul E Greenberg, 2015)

According to the Centers for Medicare & Medicaid Services, the federal agency which administers Medicaid, just over 80 million people were enrolled in the program as of January 2021. This number represents a 13.9% increase from February 2020, for a pair of programs that already represented the "largest single source of health coverage in the country." (CMS.gov, 2021) By October 2022, according to the total enrollment in these programs had increased to over 91 million (CMS.gov, 2023) .

Why mention all this?

Because in brief, Medicaid needs help.

Let's start with the question of access. "Do you see patients with Medicaid?" Now, a lot of effort has been made to make sure people do have access to facilities which accept Medicaid. In my state, Medicaid-insured patients usually rely on state-funded mental health clinics. These are clinics that are run by the state through its mental health department. There are wide-reaching efforts to provide these facilities to all communities, including both rural and urban settings. Now usually, these clinics offer what's called *wraparound services*, i.e., enough services to "wrap around" the patient. This "total package" of services includes social work, case management, in-clinic treatment, and therapy. It's a full-service modality that has been shown to help treat not only active mental health issues, but to also prevent worsening of minor mental health issues.

As I've noted elsewhere, if mental health is addressed, other issues will improve!

So certainly, there is greater access than ever before to mental health facilities which accept Medicaid. That sounds great, right?

Well, I wish we could end the chapter here, on a happy note. I'm sorry to tell you, a book titled *This Isn't Working* is not going to be jam-packed with good news. For one thing, the old adage of "if you build it, they will come" may be true for a baseball field in Dyersville, Iowa, but in health care, attendance is much less consistent. What most anyone in health care will recognize as a major roadblock to improved care is the "no-show rate," also referred to as *non-adherence*, which are both fancy terms for when a patient fails to show up for their scheduled appointment. This is especially true in my field of behavior health care, where no-show rates are reported around 30%. (Lefforge N.L., 2007) If a patient "no-shows" their appointment, that is time not being invested in their mental health care, addressing symptoms, treatments, and improving prognosis.

Keeping appointment times can be especially difficult in the economic circumstances of Medicaid patients. Severe illness, childcare, reliable transportation, and job responsibilities, while obstacles for most any person, are often especially difficult challenges for those covered by Medicaid. Compounding their difficulty, many physicians in private practices do not accept Medicaid patients, mostly due to low reimbursement rates. (Tami L. Mark, 2020)

How do clinics currently deal with no-shows? Personal reminder calls from staff and walk-in-only appointments are a couple of ways clinics improve adherence. Medicaid also covers rides to Medicaid-covered medical appointments, and clinics may try to direct patients to that resource if transportation is an issue. But truthfully? Clinics are limited in their options.

Certain things clinics cannot and should not do. No-show fees, for instance, are not allowed under the Medicaid program.

Recently, this situation was drastically improved. With the COVID-19 pandemic, the government declared a public health emergency and, among many other things, eased restrictions on telehealth visits. No-show rates improved dramatically as a direct result. A 2021 study demonstrates the significant improvement in no-show rates following the loosening of rules around virtual care. At a primary and specialty care clinic, the no-show rate for in-office visits before the pandemic was 29.8%. This number rose to 36.1% for in-office visits during the pandemic. But for telehealth visits during the pandemic, the no-show rate was only 7.9%! (Drerup, Espenschied, Wiedemer, & Hamilton, 2021)

But in the healthcare industry it tends to be two steps forward, one step (potentially) back. The eased regulations around telehealth are on thin ice. The legal conditions which allow telehealth visits were implemented as an emergency stopgap measure. The time remaining for these conditions is extremely short. Currently, the Consolidated Appropriations Act of 2023 has extended the eased regulations around telehealth out to December 2024. We can only hope these rules will be implemented in a more permanent fashion before then.

But outside of telehealth, what more can be done? And just why am I so concerned with improving non-adherence rates anyway?

In my practice, I have encountered many patients with Medicaid who struggle, even with virtual care, to adhere to their scheduled appointments. I want to talk for a minute about just how important it is to find strategies and options to help Medicaid patients meet appointments, and how missing appointments derails treatment and threatens to worsen symptoms.

Please meet Sandra. Sandra is a hypothetical patient with Medicaid.

Sandra has multiple medical issues, but what's pertinent here is she suffers from both seizures and depression. The seizures, I unfortunately could do nothing about. But over time, her depression improved.

She was enrolled in Medicaid and had come seeking care for both her depression and seizures at the academic health system. Sandra had many plates she was working hard to keep spinning. She was helping her adult daughter, both financially and in caring for her granddaughter. She was also trying to keep her job, which did not provide health care benefits. Unfortunately, due to her considerable time constraints, she often no-showed her appointments with me. I knew Sandra wanted to come, but she couldn't. So, a treatment plan that would normally take 6-10 weeks of antidepressant trial and evaluation took much longer with Sandra. Despite this, she did improve and was looking forward to brighter and better days.

But on a routine check-up with Sandra, I noticed she wasn't doing well. She said that recently, she had not been able to get to her neurologist for several follow-up visits. She had subsequently forgotten to request her anti-seizure medication. After a week when she was unable to get her medication, she had a seizure. Sandra had since re-engaged treatment with her neurologist and was stable, but due to restrictions related to her recent seizure, she was now unable to drive. This was detrimental both to her ability to work and to care for her grandchild. We spoke more, and I offered what support I could. But the writing was on the wall. No medication or supportive statements could really improve her situation. Life was hitting Sandra hard, and she was waiting for the storm to pass.

Let's meet one more patient.

His name is Jerry. Jerry is also a hypothetical patient who has Medicaid.

He came to the psychiatry resident clinic at the request of his PCP, who was urging Jerry to seek help for his severe alcohol use. Though young, Jerry's liver had substantial hepatic cirrhosis. His doctor was doing what he could to alleviate his medical issues, but the medicine Jerry most needed was to *stop drinking*. Enter the psychiatrist.

But truth be told, Jerry really, really, did not want to be in my clinic. His family had urged him to follow his PCP's instructions and address his alcoholism, and he had relented. So, there he was, sitting in front of me, with a stale scent of cigarettes and alcohol. His caring mother was at his side. I was confident I could help Jerry. The biggest question was, would he allow himself to be helped?

We completed the evaluation, set up a treatment plan, and scheduled a follow-up visit. What ensued was months of missed appointments, then calls from his family reporting that Jerry was drinking again and not taking his medications. He was also frequenting the emergency room to have his abdomen fluid drained.

Let's take a quick medical minute. Liver cirrhosis is essentially scarring of the liver. What is associated with cirrhosis is ascites (pronounced like "uh-sai-tees"), which is fluid accumulation in the abdomen. This fluid is often drained for comfort and to avoid infection, which can become very serious.

I would see Jerry on occasion, and we would resume care in my clinic briefly, only for him to disappear shortly after. Appointment slots that would have been available for more enthusiastic patients, including other Medicaid patients, were instead taken up by an empty chair.

This cycle unfortunately continued for nearly a year. Finally, Jerry realized he felt better when he took his medications and had less urge to drink excessively. On one visit, he candidly said to me, "I actually don't want to keep drinking and I don't want to die." This was an important moment for Jerry. It could herald a turnaround that would save his life. I had wondered if he would let me help him. Now it seemed a window of opportunity had opened just a crack. But this is where Jerry's story ends, at least in this book. Instead, I want to finish his story with this question: do you think he will get better if he makes his appointment times? Do you think he'll get worse if he doesn't?

Sandra and Jerry have different, yet similar problems. Sandra and Jerry need support. Sandra cannot, and Jerry will not. But they would both benefit immensely from a little more help.

Can I make a suggestion? I think what Sandra and Jerry needed was an advocate. Someone to help them make their appointments, check in on them, and even offer some counseling grounded in training.

Let me explain further. Sandra could not keep her plates spinning. She was being pulled in too many directions, and as commonly happens, her health took a backseat. But an occurrence of seizure puts Sandra out of the game, right when she needs to be the star quarterback, not on the sideline.

Jerry wouldn't. For a prolonged period, Jerry's mental health issues precluded him from seeing his alcohol use needed treatment, and he utilized expensive emergency room visits for his care. Even having experienced his moment of clarity, at the moment we left him, he had not yet escaped his self-destructive patterns. Both Sandra and Jerry need someone in their corner.

I propose what I call the "Medicaid Healthcare Advocate."

Traditionally, a medical durable power of attorney is a written assignment one makes to someone they trust (a healthcare proxy) to make healthcare decisions in the event they are unable to do so.

I propose a new character in the healthcare arena. A merging of social worker and medical personnel (a medical assistant (MA) or a licensed practical nurse (LPN)), serving as a Healthcare Advocate for a person insured with Medicaid.

Let's do an example.

Bob is having abdominal pain. Bob is meeting with his Medicaid Healthcare Advocate, or MHA, on Wednesday to check-in. In my ideal world, this can be done virtually, or even by telephone.

During their meeting, Bob mentions the abdominal pain. The MHA takes a brief history and compiles the information into an online request to Bob's primary care clinician's office to schedule an appointment. She coordinates and reports to Bob that he has an appointment in two days with the Nurse Practitioner in the Primary Care's clinic. Bob reminds his MHA that his car is not working, so the MHA also coordinates the community van to pick up Bob and take him to his appointment.

The next week, after Bob's appointment with his Primary Care's Nurse Practitioner, the MHA and Bob meet to discuss the plan reported by the clinician. The MHA relays that they are concerned Bob is having gallbladder issues and he needs an ultrasound. Bob requests more information about his gallbladder and the next steps. The MHA sends Bob an information sheet in his email.

The MHA coordinates the ultrasound appointment, again arranges transportation, and receives the ultrasound report after the completion of the scan. The MHA ensures Bob's PCP also receives the imaging report and helps coordinate a referral to a general surgeon, as the ultrasound found gallstones in the gallbladder that are the likely culprit of Bob's abdominal pain.

What ultimately results (ideally) is Bob's timely operation for his gallbladder removal. What is less likely to happen? Missed appointments, resulting in a delay of diagnosis and a worsening of symptoms, and possibly even ER visits and prolonged hospitalization from an infection in Bob's gallbladder.

Constructing a cost-benefit analysis to weigh the net cost to the Medicaid program for Bob's MHA against Bob attempting to do this on his own would, I believe, surely show a far heftier sum in the latter possibility. An average overnight hospital stay can cost $11,700 and the average salary of a medical assistant is around $38,000 (Charaba, 2023; Salary.com). With the assumption the MA would be managing multiple Medicaid recipients, I believe the scale would weigh in the favor of the MHA.

So, to close out this chapter, let's tackle the delicate subject of Medicaid patients, like Jerry, who need extra motivation.

Combining two elements already utilized in our society, I propose the concept of the Medicaid Contingency Manager, or MCM. Welfare participation already requires certain criteria to be met, such as work requirements. And existing contingency management programs for substance abuse sometimes reward patients for attending treatment and achieving negative urine drug screens. What if we combine these elements to form the MCM?

In the MCM, points are assigned for meeting certain elements. A sort of Medicaid "score" could be given to each participant. This could be based on complexity of medical issues, number of medications, and/or the number of specialist physicians. This score would serve as the foundational aspect of the patient's eligibility and benefits. Points could be awarded for making and keeping appointments and adherence to medications based on timely fills of prescriptions, which would improve the patient's Medicaid score. This could also lead to rewards. As the patient accumulates points, these points could equate to a grocery gift card, gas card, or meal card. Contingency management programs demonstrate that these kinds of rewards work. Look at the VA (Veterans Affairs). Since 2011, the U.S. Department of Veterans Affairs have used contingency management in their substance abuse clinics. Patients are rewarded with vouchers to the VA canteen where they can purchase groceries, clothing, sundries. What has resulted is 92% of the urine drug tests being negative. (Johnson, 2022)

So why stop the rewarding for substance related issues? What about Jerry who not only has a substance use issue, but also a severe medical issue related to his substance use? If Jerry received $25

Walmart gift card for keeping his appointments, filling his medications, and completing negative drug tests, would he have more motivation to put his health care as a priority? Research would suggest yes.

Alternatively, repeatedly failing to make appointments might negatively impact the score. Some may find this punitive or harsh, but some element of patient responsibility may improve outcomes, besides addressing this issue from an administrative approach.

As a mental health provider, it is disheartening to see the struggles of my patients. Patients are so happy to learn I see those covered by Medicaid. Most are eager to make appointments and receive their care. Of course, daily life carries many hurdles. But those who consistently miss appointments end up in and out of the ER or inpatient psychiatric units due to unmanaged symptoms. And when they call for help, which we are eager to give, and are still unable to show up to appointments, they take appointment slots from those who are desperate to get in. The hospital systems receive less reimbursement for ill patients who sometimes require longer hospital stays. The system is not working, and the concept of managed care to help assist has good intentions, but the reality of success is too early to say. Addressing and assisting those who struggle to make appointments with more managed care and incentives could result in a system that radically improves adherence and, consequently, health outcomes.

Does Medicaid need help? Definitely. But it's help we are capable of providing. I've thrown out a few possible solutions, but what's most important is that *something* happens. With such a large uptick of

Medicaid patients post-COVID, the current issues are only going to become more exacerbated. Remember, it will be the most vulnerable among us who will suffer if we allow the system to simply limp along. Many of my Medicaid patients are good, hardworking people who just caught some bad breaks. Let's do more to provide them with the treatment they need, psychiatric and otherwise. Because what are we doing now? Offering help and care for those in bad circumstances, but allowing those circumstances to impair the care we're offering? This isn't working.

American Psychological Association. (2020). *"Stress in America(TM) 2020: A National Mental Health Crisis"*. Retrieved from https://www.apa.org/news/press/releases/stress/2020/report-october

American Psychological Association. (2021). *"Stress in America(TM) 2021: One year later, a new wave of pandemic health concerns"*. Retrieved from https://www.apa.org/news/press/releases/stress/2021/one-year-pandemic-stress

Charaba, C. (Producer). (2023, January 12). "Infographic: How much does a hospital stay cost?". *PeopleKeep*. Retrieved from https://www.peoplekeep.com/blog/infographic-how-much-does-a-hospital-stay-cost

CMS.gov. (2021). "New Medicaid and CHIP Enrollment Snapshot Shows Almost 10 million Americans Enrolled in Coverage During the COVID-19 Public Health Emergency" [Press release]. Retrieved from https://www.cms.gov/newsroom/press-releases/new-medicaid-and-chip-enrollment-snapshot-shows-almost-10-million-americans-enrolled-coverage-during

CMS.gov. (2023, January 31). "November 2022 Medicaid & CHIP Enrollment Data Highlights". *Centers for Medicare & Medicaid Services*. Retrieved from https://www.medicaid.gov/medicaid/program-information/medicaid-and-chip-enrollment-data/report-highlights/index.html

Drerup, B., Espenschied, J., Wiedemer, J., & Hamilton, L. (Producer). (2021, December). "Reduced No-Show Rates and Sustained Patient Satisfaction of Telehealth During the COVID-19 Pandemic". *Telemedicine and e-Health*. Retrieved from http://doi.org/10.1089/tmj.2021.0002

Johnson, C. K. (Producer). (2022, September 7). "Candy, cash, gifts: How rewards help recovery from addiction". *AP News*. Retrieved from https://apnews.com/article/how-rewards-helps-recovery-from-addiction-6d11673c55fae3a413dcc5f57ca5e104

Lefforge N.L., D. B., Strada M.J. (2007). Improving session attendance in mental health and substance abuse settings: A review of controlled studies. *Behavior Therapy*, 38(31): 31-22.

Nirmita Panchal, R. K., Cynthia Cox, Rachel Garfield (Producer). (2021, February 10). "The Implications of COVID-19 for Mental Health and Substance Use". *Kaiser*

Family *Foundation*. Retrieved from
https://www.kff.org/report-section/the-implications-of-covid-19-for-mental-health-and-substance-use-issue-brief/

Paul E Greenberg, A.-A. F., Tammy Sisitsky, Crystal T Pike, and Ronald C Kessler. (2015). "The economic burden of adults with major depressive disorder in the United States (2005 and 2010)". *The Journal of Clinical Psychiatry*.

Salary.com. "Medical Assistant Salary in the United States". Retrieved from
https://www.salary.com/research/salary/benchmark/medical-assistant-salary

Tami L. Mark, P. D., M.B.A., William Parish, Ph.D., Gary A. Zarkin, Ph.D., Ellen Weber, J.D. (Producer). (2020, July 24). Comparison of Medicaid Reimbursements for Psychiatrists and Primary Care Physicians. *PsychiatryOnline.org*. Retrieved from https://doi.org/10.1176/appi.ps.202000062

Chapter Seven

Would You Like Fries With That?

In a moment of particular snarkiness one day, while typing aggressively on the hospital computer, a hematologist/oncologist stopped by my computer station and asked, "Is the psychiatrist having a bad day?" A patient's family had put me through the wringer of endless questions from which I was left wondering why they had requested my professional consult at all when they clearly believed they knew more than I did about delirium.

I responded, "Me? The psychiatrist? Sometimes I think I may just be a customer services representative with an M.D. at the end of my name." I mean, physicians do receive patient satisfaction scores that can affect their income. Already many professions depend on customer surveys for raises and even job security. But frankly we, as customers, do not always know what goes into jobs that aren't our own. Let alone the circumstance in which a patient does not receive, let's just throw this out there, a prescription for a controlled substance that they really want, from the physician, they can simply respond extremely negatively to the review, even when the physician was acting in the best interest of the patient by practicing according to guidelines.

Speaking of guidelines and expertise, as I have made clear throughout this book, I consider my career as a psychiatrist to be a life's work. It's an honor to care for and treat the people I encounter daily. But there are obstacles to my work.

So let me paint you a picture here.

Let's say your toilet is broken. You don't know what is wrong with it, but it needs to be fixed, now. You call the plumber recommended to you by your friendly neighbor, who commented that this plumber "is quick, cheap, and will get the job done."

The plumber shows up, takes a look at the toilet and states that it needs a new part. Part A. So, he says he needs to get a new Part A for you. Says it costs around $10.00 for the part, plus labor costs, and he can get the toilet repaired today. You agree and the plumber moves forward with the plan.

In this situation, you called a specialist, the plumber, who diagnosed the problem, presented the solution, and you both agreed with the plan and moved forward. This collaboration between specialist and customer is more or less the ideal.

While I appreciate a toilet is not, say, your heart, that needs to be fixed, that's even more reason to trust the expertise and training of the cardiovascular surgeon who makes a recommendation for a repair of the heart.

I bring to you my patient Janice. Janice is an amalgamation of patients I treated during residency training.

Janice is extremely anxious about her first visit but is ready to do something about her daily anxiety that affects her functioning.

I explained the diagnosis, the treatment recommendations, and asked how she felt about the plan. Janice said that she did not want to be on lots of medications but would consider the recommendations. She did ask if I could refill her lorazepam (benzodiazepine, in the same category as alprazolam, a.k.a. Xanax) for her. I counseled her on the guidelines for anxiety and the recommendations for use of lorazepam (see the "Xannies" chapter for more information). She said she wanted to think about her options, which I usually encourage. I do not expect my patients to decide in the moment if they agree with a medical plan. Janice called back the next day having decided she wanted to try the medications suggested. After a brief time, her anxiety improved, and she was stable.

Unfortunately, she called several months later reporting worsening of symptoms. During her visit, the options were explained to her. She attested that she really just wanted more lorazepam. Again, I advised that though the lorazepam could be useful to abort a panic attack, the guidelines and her response to medications would suggest simply a dose increase of her current regimen. She then stated she had spoken to her sister-in-law who advised that, in her opinion, she should just be on the lorazepam.

At this junction, after my advice was given, and in the light of her actually improving from my previous recommendations, I stated that these were my recommendations, but I would suggest she reconsider them and let us know.

I do appreciate that, if the plumber did royally mess up that toilet, one could simply be purchased later that day at a hardware store. Obviously, not the same with a heart, or any other part of the human body. No discounts or credit card rewards for a new pancreas. I am not against the idea of a second opinion. But what makes good health care difficult is when the expertise of a physician is questioned to the point that one essentially could leave a health situation without a problem solved.

Chapter Eight

The 21st Century Cures Act

A federal rule came into effect in 2021 called the Cures Act ensuring that most notes documented in a patient's chart (with minor exceptions) must be made available in real-time to a patient. The intent is to eliminate hiccups in one's medical care, so information can be readily shared between hospital systems and ensure the patient has real-time access to their own medical records.

On paper, this sounds great.

In reality, it isn't.

I was consulted to see a patient in the hospital. The patient had underlying psychiatric issues that were unstable, with new acute medical issues. I documented on the patient utilizing my standard template for inpatient consultations. This template includes assessing for psychiatric background as well as any substance concerns, which is standard for a psychiatric evaluation.

So, this gentleman, in his late 50's, was under the care of his parents, their early 80's. I received a call from the hospitalist that the patient's parents had some concerns about documentation in the chart. Somewhat perplexed, I contacted the patient's parents.

They were extremely kind and sweet, but they, with their daughter, had reviewed their son's notes on the online patient portal, and were very concerned that I had documented the patient had substance issues, when he did not.

As one who takes documentation extremely seriously, I immediately hopped on the electronic medical records to review my consultation note. I simply could not find what they were describing. All I could see was the heading in the template of 'Substance History' where I had written, "No pertinent issues at this time."

I read this with the parents on the phone. The patient's parents said they must have read it wrong and had no other questions.

Ten minutes total spent explaining my template to these extremely kind and concerned parents.

I do not think this is what the Cures Act intended.

I have since encountered so many troubling experiences with patients in the hospital having real-time access to their clinical notes. One patient who had a very difficult time understanding her severe anemia, newly discovered metastatic cancer, as well as pregnancy, utilized her access to her online portal to question every single doctor of the labs, the documentation, and treatment plan, although it had been discussed with her in real-time multiple times. What resulted were countless hours spent by the medical team trying to justify to this patient their reasoning, their documentation, and their plan.

Another instance of a patient admitted due to severe anorexia requiring medical care comes to mind. The patient utilized her daily access to her portal to review the notes, which included the calorie content of her tube feeds. which troubled her and potentially led to her tampering with her tube feeds to avoid calorie intake.

Ten minutes of my day lost checking over my consult template is clearly the least of issues being caused. I have more reservations about this act's ratio of utility versus harm in the acute care setting where a patient who is psychiatrically unstable has instant access to their medical records.

Of course, the Cures Act can't be written off as all bad. As a patient in healthcare, having the ability to quickly review and understand my medical records has such a positive aspect, especially since I can never remember the plan when I leave a doctor's office.
The Cures Act rides the line between helpful and hurtful, as so many things do.

Chapter Nine

Ask Your Doctor If This Medication Will Work for You

If you have a TV and see commercials, you have probably encountered an advertisement for one of many psychiatric medications. They all have the same thematic concept. One in particular utilizes "happy face" and "sad face" paper signs that the "patient" actor puts on her face hiding her true feelings. Then once the patient receives the psychiatric medication advertised, the sad faces become happy faces. Perfect, right?

I have to ask. Why on Earth are medications being advertised directly to consumers?

These medications are usually geared towards serious mental illness like bipolar disorder or bipolar depression, in other words, relatively rare conditions. The prevalence of bipolar disorder is 1% of the population. So why do you think these pharmaceutical companies are paying to produce and air TV advertisements?

A few years ago, one of the advertisements was actually for one of my favorite medications I prescribe. I feel my patients do well on it and have less side effects than others available in that category. (This meets my two important goals when treating someone. Good response and minimal side effects. Easier said than done).

I rarely prescribed this favorite medication of mine, until recently. Can you guess why?

If insurance does not cover this medication, it can cost *$1400 a month*. It recently became available in a generic form, but when brand name was the only option, $1400 a month was not feasible for most of my patients and their insurance formularies. Hence, the advertisements! Once a medication can be made into a generic, you rarely see advertisements for it.

So here comes the board game I will call "Healthcare Hazards." On one side of the game, you have the insurance company. The other side, the pharmaceutical company. In the middle, the physician trying to manage the patient's symptoms. Patient comes to clinic. Sees add for fancy medication "Smileagain." Doctor tells patient "Smileagain" is rarely covered by insurance, and, also, is not indicated (that is, recommended based on treatment guidelines for a certain condition) for their diagnosis of simple depression. Patient insists they wish to try medication.

Doctor reviews risk and benefits with patient who expresses understanding but again insists on trying medication. What ensues is likely a long conversation between the insurance company and pharmacy which requires paperwork, called a prior authorization, to be filled out by the physician, at no charge, so the physician can attest why the patient needs this $1400 per month medication, when one chemically very similar costs $30 a month.

Physicians deal with this frequently.

Remember the chapter with the plumber who made a recommendation for Part A that needed to be fixed? Does the customer of the plumber question whether Part A is the best or should Part B, which costs $2 less than Part A be used? Does the painter use the best option they have for the customer in the color requested, while being mindful of the customer's budget?

Or even this one! Does the surgeon tell the patient which type of suture is going to be used for the surgery and why? Probably not.

Chapter Ten

Where Have All the Psychiatrists Gone?

In a *New York Times* article from 1982, the author reported the following:" From 1970 to 1980 the percentage of medical students drawn to psychiatry fell from above 11 percent to less than half that proportion" (Nelson, 1982).

In the forty years since this article was published, the situation has not much improved. In 2012, it was reported that 46% of psychiatrists were age 55 or older, compared with 35% of other practicing physicians (Caccavale, Reeves, & Wiggins, 2012).

So how could we not expect a shortage of psychiatrists in 2023? Luckily, the last few years have shown a strong interest in graduating medical students who are pursuing careers in psychiatry. But until the shift regulates, it is not unexpected that the field will rely on "mid-level practitioners" or physician assistant or advanced practitioners, such as nurse practitioners, to help carry the weight of patients needing help.

It is important to reinforce these practitioners with quality education and the importance of practice guidelines.

Take a look at when this can go wrong.

In May 2022, the US Department of Justice initiated an investigation of the mental health startup Cerebral due to prescriptions of medications Xanax and Adderall, used for the treatment of ADHD. After a 30-minute video call, one could be given a diagnosis of ADHD and a prescription for Adderall, a schedule II-controlled substance (There are five schedules for controlled substances, with I being the most controlled. For reference, heroin is schedule I). The prescribing of these medications through a video call became possible as regulations loosened due to the COVID-19 pandemic, including those regulations requiring in-person visits prior to prescribing of controlled substances.

While the loosening of regulations helped those in need access their physicians virtually during the pandemic, it is not a surprise to anyone living in this world that a business idea may come forward to take advantage of a necessary arrangement. And furthermore, that an arrangement that has good intent ends up failing miserably. Call it greed, or whatever you wish, the issue is that if we do not restrict access the correct way, we risk hurting the populations we are trying to help by flooding them with powerful, and unnecessary, drugs.

Caccavale, J., Reeves, M. J. L., & Wiggins, J. (2012). *The impact of psychiatric shortage on patient care and mental health policy: The silent shortage that can no longer be ignored*. Retrieved from

Nelson, B. (1982). Psychiatry's Anxious Years: Decline in Allure; As a Career Leads to Self-Examination. *The New York Times*. Retrieved from https://www.nytimes.com/1982/11/02/science/psychiatry-s-anxious-years-decline-allure-career-leads-self-examination.html

Chapter Eleven

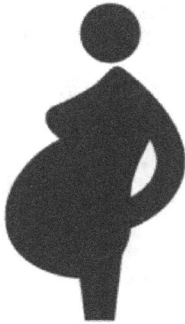

Women's Mental Health

"Hey, it's Dr. Adams. You got a second?"

This was my personal OB-GYN calling during my clinic. He had a question about a patient and needed assistance. One of his patients, age 36, was post-partum and had told Dr. Adams that she was repeatedly having suicidal thoughts when driving on a specific part of the highway. He had tried her on an antidepressant, but it did not seem to be working, and needed recommendations.

I made several, including medications and therapy options, but most importantly, safety recommendations.

I said, "She should not drive, should be monitored by family, and should call the clinic or go to the ER if suicidal thoughts increase in frequency or severity."

"Thank you so much," Dr. Adams said. "If you have some availability to get her in to clinic, can you help?"

Women's Mental Health.

Women's mental health warrants a whole book on its own. But since we don't have a whole book to focus on the subject, this chapter will focus on one group of women whose mental health struggles are in major need of attention. That group is women during pregnancy and immediately after, in what we call the *postpartum* period. There is a specific field of psychiatry which covers this group of women, and it's called *perinatal psychiatry*.

Let's start our discussion with a high-risk case for postpartum depression. Let's start with Alice. Alice is loosely based on a patient treated during my residency training.

Alice is a 42-year-old female, with four children, ages 2 through 8. She has a significant other, who is the father of her youngest two children. One of her children comes with special challenges. Her 4-year-old son has recently been diagnosed with moderate autism. He requires interventions including physical, occupational, and speech therapy, with appointments several times a week. Her two oldest children are often with their father, but Alice has shared custody.

Alice herself has a severe mood disorder. Diagnosing this mood disorder has turned out to be difficult. She experiences manic episodes—which, by definition, are periods of erratic behavior—with a decreased need for sleep, impulsivity, and being more talkative, to name some of the criteria. Clinically, she has had affective instability (aka mood swings), difficulty controlling anger, impulsivity, and unstable relationships. These latter symptoms are often seen in borderline personality disorder (BPD). She has several traits but does not seem to meet all the criteria for BPD.

Though Alice's diagnosis is not 100% clear, treating her symptoms has proven beneficial. She is not requiring hospitalization, she reports adherence to her medication regimen, and feels she is experiencing less mood shifts.

All these factors combine to put Alice at extreme risk for serious postpartum depression.

As I've mentioned before, the impact of effectively treating a mental illness does not end with the patient themselves. The positive effects ripple out to others in that patient's life. When someone with mental illness is treated and the symptoms improve, those around that person can have a direct benefit from this improvement. It's what I like to call the "ripples reward." Alice doing better will be a success by itself. But the "ripples reward" was knowing that her children may benefit from her improvement.

I have met Alice's children on many occasions. Alice often had to bring her children to her appointment. It's generally not preferable for a patient to bring their children to their psychiatry appointment, as sensitive information may be discussed. Obviously, the confidentiality of the appointment is gone. And I must censor myself slightly to avoid words and questions that the children may pick up on. For instance, Alice may need to discuss instances of suicidal ideation. This is a raw and difficult area of someone's life to broach in the best of circumstances, and much more difficult when we're speaking in code. But because of this, I got to meet her children and learn their faces. I remember seeing the stress and fatigue in their young faces and hoping that if Alice felt a little better, maybe this would improve.

There were hiccups. One time Alice came with her daughter wearing an arm cast. I immediately asked what happened. Alice said, "Oh, I wasn't watching, and she closed the door to the bedroom on her finger. It was just hanging off!" Since then, the girl's doctor had been forced to upgrade her simple hand cast into a full arm cast, since being just three years old, she frequently banged her hand on walls and surfaces, slowing her healing process.

Moving past the mental image of this poor girls' finger dangling from her hand, I latched onto the first part of her sentence: "*I wasn't watching.*"

Now trust me that I recognize children cannot feasibly be monitored by a parent or guardian 100% of the time. But taken together with Alice's condition, I had some concern. As with any patient, and by the requirements by law, I am always aware of any story or account that is told to me that is concerning for child abuse or neglect. Fun exercise, google your state and the terms 'child abuse reporting'. What you will find is (hopefully) a summary of who by your state's laws needs to report any situation which is concerning for a child's well-being, specifically abuse and neglect. Also, it will include elder abuse reporting requirements. Spoiler: it's *everyone*. Every citizen has a duty to report observations that point to child abuse.

I asked some questions about the injury and came away feeling assured that it was just a freak accident that left this child in a full arm cast. However, it was clear that Alice was overwhelmed and needed help.

After that appointment, Alice disappeared. She didn't show up to her scheduled appointments, and she did not return phone calls from the clinic to make new ones. For six months, we heard nothing.

Finally, Alice called the clinic. She stated she had stopped her medications and wanted to be seen in clinic; she was pregnant.

I made sure we got her into clinic the next day. I came into the appointment feeling a bit concerned. In the past, when Alice was on less medication, or even a different regimen, her mental status had not been good. She had been extremely irritable, had not been caring for herself, and had even struggled to care for her children. Coming off her medication was going to come with difficult challenges, and frankly, I was concerned as to her ability to meet these challenges.

Alice, on the other hand, came into the appointment full of excitement and ready to talk about the future. "I can't believe I'm pregnant at my age!" she said.

I wanted to catch up, as it had been six months.

A lot had happened, other than this pregnancy. One night a few months prior, her significant other and father of her two youngest children had struck her, in front of the children. She had called the police, and because of concerns about the welfare of the children, the two youngest were placed in foster care and the two oldest were placed with their father.

Alice was understandably torn up by this but was determined to get her children back. She had started working at a fast-food joint; having a job was a requirement by the judge to show she was ready to have her children in her custody.

While following her story, I had a pressing question I needed answered.

I asked who the father of the baby was.

Alice, who I have known for years, started laughing. She had caught on to the gist of my question immediately. "Oh my gosh, Dr. K, it's not him!" She had met someone new and incidentally became pregnant.

Next, we reviewed the risks of the medications she had previously taken. I told her one, lithium, has a known risk of possible cardiac issues in the fetus. She was on a low dose, and I counseled her that in most cases, we do continue this medication, as discontinuing could lead to destabilization of her mental status. Alice said she understood the risks, but still wanted to be off the medication. She was on another medication considered safe in pregnancy that could keep her mood stabilized on its own. We came up with a plan she was comfortable with and made her follow-up visit.

I am going to be extremely delicate as I move forward with this discussion.

And maybe I'll even put a disclaimer.

I believe women who wish to have children and become a mother should be able to do so. But I also provide care for women to ensure they are able to mentally withstand the stress of their lives, including caring for children. I also believe that children should be cared for in the best way that is feasibly possible.

Alice had truly improved from our initial visit. She did not berate her children in front of me, as she did in those early visits. I would watch their faces, weary and often tear-stained, and attest that I would do my best to improve this situation to the best of my abilities.

But Alice had a lot on her plate. Remember that image I described in the 'Xannies' chapter of the donkey carrying the cart with too much of a load? That image applied to Alice.

One of her children required intense therapy of multiple disciplines. This was several appointments a week with the hopes that he would meet more milestones in regard to his speech and physical capabilities.

Alice had three other children, and now, was alone, as she had no contact with her previous significant other who had physically abused her.

The gentleman in her life she met at work. She said he was very supportive of the pregnancy, and she was hopeful of this relationship.

Two days later, Alice called the clinic extremely upset. She had lost the pregnancy.

I saw her in clinic a few weeks after this. She expressed gratitude of the miracle that was the pregnancy but expressed some relief, stating she knew it was probably too much for her.

To conclude Alice's story, she had completed the requirements from the judge and was awaiting a court date to solidify reunification, i.e., she was getting her kids back. She was extremely happy, and as I helped her see, proud of herself. She had gone through a horrible experience and come out the other side. But Alice's story is not unique.

I want you to meet one other person. Her name is Catherine. Same disclaimer, not actually one person, but a culmination of many real and case study patients.

Catherine is a 27-year-old woman who has struggled with cannabis and alcohol abuse for several years. She has a significant trauma history, marked by sexual abuse as a child. She is recently married, but even that stability is on tenuous ground, as she has a history of infidelity. She expressed consistent fear her husband was having an affair.

So, it's in this environment that Catherine, also, was wanting to have a child.

Unfortunately, Catherine had limited medical care due to a lack of insurance, and she was unwilling to use community medical centers and mental health centers that offer care to the uninsured. This further escalated my concern about her ability to take over her own healthcare. With some urging, she was able to purchase health insurance through the health insurance marketplace. She then established care with a primary care physician and a gynecologist. It was at these appointments it came to light she was not ovulating, i.e., releasing eggs from her ovary so they could be positioned for conception.

At a follow-up visit, Catherine stated she had completed labs for her primary care physician to assess her hormones. She said her physician expressed hope that she could become pregnant but did not recommend medication to help Catherine ovulate until she could demonstrate sobriety.

At the time, she was using inhaled cannabis 5 times a day, and drinking 2-3 bottles of wine a night. This level of cannabis and alcohol use would put any fetus at risk of alcohol related intellectual disability (fetal alcohol syndrome), substance withdrawal at birth, and numerous other medical issues, not to mention the risks to the mother.

Catherine, on several occasions, had attempted to overcome her abuse of cannabis and alcohol. She wanted sobriety but was having difficulty getting there. She had refused recommendations for rehabilitation, stating "it would interfere with Mark's competition dates." Mark, her husband, was in competitive cycling, and she did not want to affect his upcoming races.

Her general physician had clear reason to be concerned, but I imagine some could be concerned, at this point in Catherine's story, about whether her reproductive rights are being respected. So, let's take a quick look at Catherine's situation from both a medical and a legal perspective.

According to the Guttmacher Institute, an organization with focus on reproductive health and rights, as of January 1st, 2022, twenty-four states consider substance abuse during pregnancy to be child abuse under civil child-welfare statutes. Three states even consider it grounds for involuntary commitment to a mental health or substance abuse treatment facility. (Guttmacher Institute, 2022)

This sounds scary, but I only bring it up to point out the seriousness of combining pregnancy and substance abuse and explain why a doctor will be so hesitant to enable the combination. If a woman is pregnant, wishes to keep it, and suffers from addiction, she absolutely has options. ACOG, the American College of Obstetricians and Gynecologists, offer several articles and guidelines on their website outlining how their professions feel about this very issue. In particular, they are firmly against criminal or civil penalties, including incarceration or involuntary commitment, in cases where women with substance abuse issues seek obstetrical care. (American College of Obstetricians and Gynecologists, 2008) ACOG recommends referring women who are pregnant with active substance abuse issues to treatment facilities that can help.

Finding these treatment facilities is, of course, its own challenge.

Very few drug treatment facilities accept pregnant women; those that do are rarely affordable and do not provide childcare. As of 2010, only nineteen states have drug treatment programs that accept pregnant women (Guttmacher Institute, 2022). ACOG's guideline report ends with the recommendation that the development of more comprehensive substance abuse programs should be considered, ones that can be accessible, effective, and without legal ramifications.

That's great, but like, is this really going to happen?

I know I shouldn't be pessimistic, because there has been growth in the development of programs for people with substance abuse issues, but **IT IS NOT and WILL NEVER BE ENOUGH.**

So, until these programs can be widely available, what I can give most people is a little education and do my best to encourage sobriety in their prenatal period. Which brings us back to Catherine.

She had made great effort to cut back on both cannabis and alcohol. But unfortunately, due to increased stress at home, and availability of cannabis at her workplace, she is struggling to reach that point. I do recall one significant point during a follow-up visit with Catherine that I think is worth sharing. It was soon after she had first mentioned her wish to conceive. All of her physicians, me included, had expressed concern about the degree of her substance use and the risks associated, both for her and her baby. She responded, "Just because I have mental illness, I shouldn't have a baby?"

Of course, this was not the message I, nor her other physicians would want her to take away.

But then what are we saying?

Just as an oncologist would make recommendations for someone with a high risk of lung cancer not to smoke, or a cardiologist would make recommendations for someone at risk from a heart attack to reduce salt and exercise, Catherine's primary care physician, OB-GYN physician, and myself were making recommendations for someone with substance use disorder who was wanting to have a baby, a physiological miracle that puts large amounts of stress on a woman's body.

For a related topic, I want to briefly touch on one subject that I became so intimately involved in from my own experience: breastfeeding. I want to share a very unique story I encountered that I think highlights where our society strives to do well but misses the mark.

I said earlier that if we care for the new mother, we are essentially caring for the child in return. And in the postpartum period, feeding is an almost immediate care that can become an extreme stress for the new mother.

A good friend from medical school introduced me to a social media group for new mothers who were also physicians focused on breastfeeding. I will say, I found this group more stressful than helpful. The number of postings, and the uniqueness of each woman's struggles, were overwhelming for a new mother. I came to rarely check the postings. But one day, the "mute this group for 30 days" option on the group settings had expired, and I came across a posting that caught my eye.

A woman was sharing her breastfeeding journey. But her post was unlike others I had read. The woman was struggling to get her 2-month-old child to latch, and it didn't take being a psychiatrist to sense her desperation.

She went on to list all the things she had tried: The number of lactation consultants, the visit to the doctors to ensure the baby did not have a tongue-tie. It went on and on. She pointed out that the baby was starting to lose weight due to her continued attempts to breastfeed with a poor latch. She talked about starting to feel detached from her baby, feeling like a failure, and having daily crying episodes. And at the end, as best from my memory as I can recall, she said something very akin to: "I just don't think I can do this anymore."

As a psychiatrist, I was alarmed. These were clear signs of postpartum depression, maybe even suicidal ideation. But since this was an online community of medical professionals, I expected that she would receive empathetic support rooted in strong knowledge of the pitfalls of postpartum depression. As one does, I went to the comments. What I saw was a kick in the gut.

I will say kindly, half of these comments were similar to, "hang in there, momma." There were few others like this.

One woman very strongly pointed out to these other physicians, "I think we need to be concerned about the original poster's words and provide support. To the original poster, please know you have tried what you can, but it is time to make sure your baby is fed, with breastmilk or formula, whatever it needs to be."

I was pleased to see others supporting this post and providing their contact information for the original poster to reach out to them to talk offline.

The other comments littered throughout were less understanding: "You need to do better. There's a reason he isn't latching. You just need to find the reason."

Another was "don't give up because please remember: Breast is Best."

For some background, the "Breast is Best" campaign is widely supported by international health organizations, like the World Health Organization. It supports the idea that babies have shown to do best if they receive breastmilk during the first 6 months of life. This is great. Sounds ideal.

But what are we doing to those who struggle with providing the ideal situation, giving breastmilk to the baby? I know how my argument could look. I am negating a campaign that is only suggesting and encouraging that women should try to breastfeed. I get this. I see situations frequently where women still shrug off this option despite its obvious benefits. In some ways, the campaign still has work to do. I will see able women in my clinic or in the hospital who, when asked if they plan to breastfeed, quickly say no. Their reasons? Some will say they tried in the past and were unsuccessful. Others actually avoid answering the question altogether.

So again, I understand the campaign's intent, but just like with anything, a well-meaning campaign of encouragement can be twisted to a doctrine of intense pressure that sensitive, hormonal women, in the delicate postpartum period, can immerse themselves in, as in the case above, to the point that the safety of the baby and the woman could be in question.

Breastfeeding comes with obstacles. While much less costly and more "recall-resistant" than formula, breastfeeding makes sizable demands on the mother's energy and time. Using premade formula or mixing powder in water can be quicker and help meet a baby's needs.

As a society and medical community, to help those I believe to be most vulnerable in our world — children —we need to take better care of our women. Addressing prenatal health care, including mental health care, with collaborative care between a primary care physician, OB-GYN, and a psychiatrist is a start.

This model will help serve those in peri-partum and postpartum periods as well.

Let's dive into those.

We discussed collaborative care earlier in the context of the primary care setting. The concept we'll look at now is much the same, but in the obstetrical clinic.

Imagine Dr. Adams, my personal OB-GYN from the beginning of this chapter, did not have to call his personal patient who happens to be a psychiatrist to make sure he was on the right track with the postpartum patient.

In an ideal situation I, the psychiatrist, would be sitting in that clinic available to see the patient myself immediately after her postpartum visit with Dr. Adams. Psychiatric clinics primarily focused on the perinatal period exist in larger cities. These clinics keep clinic availability open and correspondence with referring OB-GYNs as a priority, so the time between referral and clinic visit is kept at a minimum. The alternative, as discussed in an earlier chapter, is that Dr. Adams would keep a running list of patients he would like to be reviewed by me. He would coordinate with a nurse liaison, who would communicate to me each patient, their depression and anxiety scores, and any pertinent information. I would then relay recommendations based on the information given. This works, so far as it goes, but I want to reiterate that the psychiatrist sitting in place in the OB-GYN office is the most ideal real-time care that could be offered.

Of course, we again face the roadblock of a limited number of psychiatrists available for such a position. Also, while I imagine most OB-GYNs, if asked if they could fill up a psychiatrists' day with patients would answer emphatically with a pronounced "YES!", the overhead of a psychiatrist with open clinic time could be cost preventative for a private practice OB-GYN clinic.

Luckily, CMS, the Center for Medicare and Medicaid Services, which is part of the Department of Health and Human Services (HHS), has created billing codes that can be used for the collaborative care model for behavioral health integration (Jeongeun, 2003). Not having proper billing codes prevented earlier adoption of the collaborative care model, because knowing who was going to pay who is obviously an integral part of making medicine happen. Notwithstanding the roadblock of the limited supply of psychiatrists, I think in the future we will see psychiatrists much more readily taking part in specialty clinics, including obstetrical clinics.

Another concept to consider is one common in other countries outside of America: the post-partum center.

In Korea, this practice is referred to as *sanhujori*, and the centers themselves are called *sanhujoriwon* (*Jeongeun, 2003*). Historically, this was care provided to the mother and infant by immediate family, so the new mother is allowed time to rest and recuperate, from a week to a month(Yeoungjung & Mira, 2012). But with changing society, this has changed to external locations focused on total care of the new mother. This includes childcare, nutrition, rest, and even massages. One study showed that in 2012, about half of the female population in Korea had used a sanhujoriwon after childbirth.

These centers do not come without some concerns. In fact, the rapid growth of these centers resulted in some centers being ill-equipped, and these had to be closed (Hyun, 2000).

Another concern posed, especially for the American health care system, is who will pay for this, and how much would it cost? Ideally, health insurance companies would consider some coverage as a preventative care measure. The early care of a postpartum woman could reduce postpartum hospitalization, clinic care, and especially mental health complications.

Regardless of cost, it's clear the American healthcare system must do more to guard women's mental health if they're to avoid the most dangerous pitfalls of postpartum depression. We must add nuance to our narratives about the 'job description' of motherhood to create space for constructive outcomes for less-than-ideal situations. And we must open up difficult discussions about readiness for motherhood, because the worst outcomes for both mother and child are almost unthinkable.

While nothing in this world is completely avoidable, especially in the case of the human body and brain, I truly believe if the mental health care of women in these stages improved, the ripples of these efforts would be vast.

American College of Obstetricians and Gynecologists. (2008). *At-Risk Drinking and Illicit Drug Use: Ethical Issues in Obstetric and Gynecologic Practice.* Paper presented at the ACOG Committee Opinion No. 422.

Guttmacher Institute. (2022). Substance Abuse During Pregnancy. Retrieved from https://www.guttmacher.org/state-policy/explore/substance-use-during-pregnancy?msclkid=ded9e65eafb811ec918dd681a35562c6

Hyun, S.-C. (2000). A study on the realities and improvements of postpartum care centers in Korea. *Master's Dissertation in Kyung-Hee University*, 1-95.

Jeongeun, K. (2003). Survey on the programs of Sanhujori centers in Korea as the traditional postpartum care facilities. *Women & Health*, 38.32 (32): 107-117.

Yeoungjung, K., & Mira, C. (2012). A Study on the Change of Postpartum Care in Korea. *Asian Cultural Studies*, 26:217-240.

Chapter Twelve

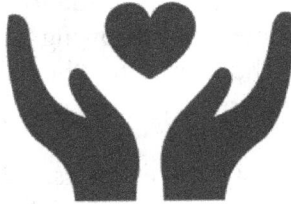

Help the Helpers

We break
We bend
With hand in hand
When hope is gone
Just hang on
Hang on

Miller/Rosenworcel/Pisapia
Guster "Hang On"

In a famous scene from the 1996 movie *Jerry Maguire*, Jerry, played by Tom Cruise pleads with his athlete client, played by Cuba Gooding, Jr., to "help me help you." This quote has long resonated with me as a healthcare provider. Whether it an uncooperative patient, or my computer failing me, I sometimes blurt out, "help me help you!" In a day where so many factors must come together for me to deliver care at a high standard, sometimes throwing my hands up in the air, begging the world to "help me help you" allows me to reset, and get to the next point I need to get to.

Over the last three years, the worldwide pandemic stressed our system. Well, 'stressed'—this is an understatement. And for all that time, our healthcare workers have been at the eye of the hurricane.

The other day I was documenting my notes on a nursing station computer on the hospital floor. I was seated next to two nurses, both familiar to me. (Which actually is a bit of a rarity recently. Between the influx of travelling nurses, and nurses vacating the hospital for various reasons, it was nice to see two familiar faces).

One nurse was speaking about recent deaths on the floor. She turned to me and said, "I wasn't supposed to be so familiar with body bags."

She spoke about a nurse who had been with the hospital for a long time but had recently decided to leave her employment. Her reason? Her father had passed from COVID-19 right on the floor she worked. Both the intensity of the pandemic and the personal loss together was just too much. I certainly could never judge her. *Can you?*

The toll the job of medical caregiver can take on one's psychological wellbeing can be extreme in the best of times. Further, there can even be trepidation in even seeking help on the mental health side.

To illustrate, I received a call late in the evening from a colleague one night. The call in itself was not unusual, as we shared many mutual patients. But the timing and the content of this call was very unusual.

This colleague, we'll call him Dr. A, is a well-informed physician. And he was calling with a very specific question. He had been reading on a social media group about seeking mental health as a physician and the possible issues that could arise from this. In particular, he was concerned about licensing. See, when a physician is getting licensed to practice in most states, they must answer several questions pertaining to their qualifications, and this includes their soundness of mind. About 90 percent of state licensing applications include at least one question about a physician's mental health, and some even ask questions about past diagnoses, such as depression or anxiety, that may have occurred before medical school (Kayla Behbahani & Thompson, 2020).

Dr. A had taken an interest in his family past and having learned some difficult information, he felt he wanted to see a therapist. But Dr. A wasn't calling me to ask for recommendations or to discuss the sort of treatment he might benefit from. His question was, "Will this affect my licensing?"

I assured Dr. A he was fine. The state licensing questions, while addressing mental health, do tend to ask if these mental health issues would affect the physician from practicing safely. I stated that learning about multi-generational trauma and processing this with a therapist would likely allow him to continue to see his patients in a safe and healthy environment. After talking with him briefly, he laughed slightly and said, "I can only imagine the calls you are getting these days."

I should note, I have fielded many calls like this since the pandemic started. The three years' post-pandemic have highlighted, in the brightest possible fluorescent ink, the mental support our healthcare workers need--and deserve. The pandemic started with health care workers being lauded as heroes, the 7pm clanking of pans at shift change, and Air Force flyovers. But the atmosphere quickly changed to one of disbelief, paranoia, treatment refusals, and physical threats and attacks. Combined with the relentless hours demanded of an acute pandemic, and we are seeing the burnout in health care workers—and the effects on our quality of care. The dwindling of nurses and physicians as our health care workers quit the workforce should make the world nervous. Physicians are growing weary of burnout assessments. Doing nothing about burnout but talk about it is just causing more burnout. As the pandemic showed, hospitals have a breaking point. And if the health care workers are not well, then how can they help the unwell?

Healthcare workers were already in an incredibly stressful environment to begin with. In a study published in the American Journal of Psychiatry over 15 years before the pandemic, authors found that the suicide rate among male physicians to be, distressingly, 1.41 times higher than the general male population (Schernhammer & Colditz, 2004). And among female physicians, the relative rate was even more pronounced — 2.27 times greater than the general female population. These tragic statistics speak of a work environment which is maximally stressful even in the best of times.

And we are not in the best of times. In fact it's clear, at this point, that the COVID-19 pandemic has spawned its own secondary pandemic, like the aftershock of an earthquake. But instead of a pandemic of a biological nature, it is a pandemic of a mental health nature. And it is hospital workers who are being affected.

Recent research is finding nurses are at an even greater risk of suicidal thoughts since the pandemic began. A survey from November 2021 revealed nurses were reporting increased suicidal thoughts (Kelsey et al., 2021).

In an article highlighting the stress of healthcare workers from the pandemic published in *The Atlantic* in November 2021, nurses describe themselves to the author as "bone-weary, depressed, irritable" (Yong, 2021). They're "constantly on the verge of tears, or prone to snapping at colleagues and patients." These intolerable conditions have consequences; I U.S. Bureau of Labor Statistics estimates that the health-care sector has lost nearly half a million workers since February 2020 (bls.gov, 2023). And for those who chose to stay, the environment of COVID naysayers and overwhelming fatigue taxed the workforce. Not to ignore the terrifying increase in violence towards healthcare workers, which we will talk more about a little later. At one facility, panic buttons were dispersed to nursing staff as the hospital system had seen assaults triple from the year 2019 to 2020 (Hollingsworth & Schultes, 2021).

Many articles have been written about the changing landscape of healthcare workers in the context of the pandemic. All refer to the same drastic flip from idolization to condemnation. We began with a couple months of military flyovers, community food donations and change of shift clapping. What transpired for the rest of the pandemic was medical doubt, entitlement, and aggression. Countless methods to improve recruitment and retention are in play. But will they work?

While attention on the pandemic and its' consequences on the healthcare worker is contemporary, the struggle of the healthcare worker is not. Their struggle continues whether you see them or not.

There are now movements to stop calling it burnout and move the discussion towards the term 'wellness.' Physicians, nurses, and all healthcare professionals want what I think most workers want: acknowledgement, respect, and dignity.

Signs now posted around the hospital reiterate that harm to a healthcare worker is a serious crime. Right here in my city, a physician, caring for a man with COVID-19, became the online target of a so-called religious group. The wife of the COVID patient demanded her husband receive a higher dose of the steroid, budesonide. A doctor was then making the rounds on the Internet with claims that inhaled budesonide was a "silver bullet" which could cure COVID-19 in 100% of cases. Today, we have seen that the drug only provides "mild benefits" when administered in COVID's early stages (Landhuis, 2022). In this patient's case, in intensive care and struggling to breathe on a ventilator, this unverified treatment was more likely to whittle down his already-thin chances. The physician chose to treat the patient to medical guidelines and his considerable expertise. Unfortunately, this man passed away, and an angry online commenter "doxed" the physician which, in Internet parlance, means releasing his private information in a public forum. The patient's evangelical religious group protested loudly outside the hospital, amplifying the situation. For months, this physician lived in fear that his family or himself might be attacked. And this was no idle fear.

A recent shooting occurred at an outpatient orthopedic clinic in a nearby city. The patient blamed the physician for his continuing back pain following a surgery. He shot the physician, another physician, a receptionist, and another patient before taking his own life. Reading that again in the most simple of text begs attention. Is it sustainable that we thanklessly work our physicians and other health care personnel until they collapse, and thank them with the horrible violence and the threat of violence? What do we expect our health care system to look like in ten years under these heartbreaking conditions? This isn't working.

I remember my first COVID room. As a psychiatrist, I did not foresee how frequently I would gown and enter a COVID-19 room during the pandemic. But COVID-related delirium was ramping up and I had been consulted to evaluate the patient. Of course, my hospital colleagues were already far too familiar with the stepped-up PPE (Personal

Protective Equipment) and safety procedures around rooms housing COVID patients. For me, the feeling was extremely new. Although I was following a path laid down by my colleagues, this moment still came very early in the pandemic. It was before vaccines, and it was before we had reliable data about treatment. I wondered what I was exposing myself to, but more importantly, I wondered what I would be exposing my family to. My daughter was then only two years old. If I got sick, would she in turn contract this strange new disease, about which was so much was still unknown? I felt my face flushing. I thought about my parents. They live in the same city. We knew even then older patients were more strongly impacted. Was I putting them in danger? I stood outside the room, my eyes minimally visible behind the shields and PPE. I took a second and attempted a deep breath through my tightly-fastened N-95. I took a shallow breath, mumbled the beginning of a prayer my parents taught me and which they relied on in times of difficulty, and entered the room. I had taken an oath, I was there to help, and in an unprecedented time of my life, the call to help was blaring, and there was no mute button.

In previous chapters, I've shared hopeful notions to repair this broken system. I believe part of provoking constructive discussion about these issues is not just pointing out problems but jumpstarting the journey to solutions. While I prefer to stay optimistic in my thoughts, beliefs, and actions, I feel I cannot reach that point with this chapter. This entire book is opining that the mental health system, and with it, several elements of our health system are broken. But I will say this.

Our medical and mental systems are surely struggling, but they are what we have. And who keeps this system churning, and more importantly, keeps our citizens alive is our healthcare workers. Not so long ago, I was travelling overseas, and the flight company workers went on strike two days before my return home! Thankfully, some agreement was met with the company workers and the strike ended, much to my relief. Clearly, had the strike carried on, my travel plans (and credit card) would have been affected by an unplanned prolongation of my trip. But I would be alive.

Healthcare workers have historically only dipped their toe into labor actions such as walk-outs and strikes. They are more aware than anyone that labor actions in the health sector can have health costs for patients, and there is no one health care workers care more about than their patients. Thus, these few labor actions usually do not last long, and usually come with mixed reviews. [[More Than 7,000 (Otterman & Piccoli, 2023) Nurses Go on Strike at Two NYC Hospitals - The New York Times (nytimes.com)]] This leaves many health care workers without recourse as their work conditions become intolerable.

While unions and organizing of physicians and healthcare workers continues to evolve, I suppose I leave this chapter with an image I will not forget.

During COVID, the hospital was closed to visitors, which resulted in a surprisingly quiet and orderly hospital. Elevators were quick to catch, hallways and seating areas were empty, and workers moved swiftly from room to room. On this day I stopped for a moment outside the COVID hallway. For some reason, at that moment I wanted to remember what I saw. I looked down the hall, each hospital room anchored with PPE waiting to be used. Yellow gowns were stacked in packaging, brown bags with names scribbled held each worker's mask and shield. They hung on shelves in the PPE "don and doffing" station. While a room marked for contact isolation due to an infectious diagnosis is common on the hospital floor, seeing a whole hallway of yellow gowns waiting to be donned stopped me in my tracks. Then I saw a physician I knew, standing at her station and putting on her PPE. I noticed she was moving slowly, fatigued from the day. She put on her armor and glanced down the hallway towards me. Even seeing only her eyes, peering through the slit formed by her face shield and mask, I could see the pain she was feeling.

Even today, revisiting the memory, I sometimes have to pause. I don't have enough words to convey the appreciation our healthcare workers deserve. To those who have died trying to care for those who were sick, a domestic martyrdom not seen in this country in maybe 100 years; for those who felt the calling to medicine had quelled, and their purpose was elsewhere; and for those who have stayed, weathered and battered but willing to heed the call, I say: thank you, my friends.

And to my reader, I say: our system *does not work* without the healthcare worker.

bls.gov. (2023). *The Employment Situation*. Retrieved from https://www.bls.gov/news.release/pdf/empsit.pdf.

Hollingsworth, H., & Schultes, G. (Producer). (2021, September 29). Health workers once saluted as heroes now get threats. *AP News*. Retrieved from https://apnews.com/article/coronavirus-pandemic-business-health-missouri-omaha-b73e167eba4987cab9e58fdc92ce0b72

Kayla Behbahani, & Thompson, A. (2020). Why don't doctors seek mental health treatment? They'll be punished for it. *The Washington Post*. Retrieved from https://www.washingtonpost.com/outlook/2020/05/11/mental-health-doctors-covid/

Kelsey, E. A., West, C. P., Cipriano, P. F., Peterson, C., Satele, D., Shanafelt, T., & Dyrbye, L. N. (2021). Suicidal ideation and attitudes toward help seeking in US nurses relative to the general working population. *AJN The American Journal of Nursing, 121*(11), 24-36.

Landhuis, E. (2022). These Are the Latest COVID Treatments. *Scientific American*.

Otterman, S., & Piccoli, S. (Producer). (2023, January 9). Nurses Go on Strike at 2 New York City Hospitals. *The New York Times*. Retrieved from https://www.nytimes.com/2023/01/09/nyregion/nurses-strike-nyc-hospitals.html

Schernhammer, E. S., & Colditz, G. A. (2004). Suicide rates among physicians: a quantitative and gender assessment (meta-analysis). *American Journal of Psychiatry, 161*(12), 2295-2302.

Yong, E. (2021). Why Health-Care Workers are Quitting in Droves. *The Atlantic*. Retrieved from https://www.theatlantic.com/health/archive/2021/11/the-mass-exodus-of-americas-health-care-workers/620713/

Chapter Thirteen

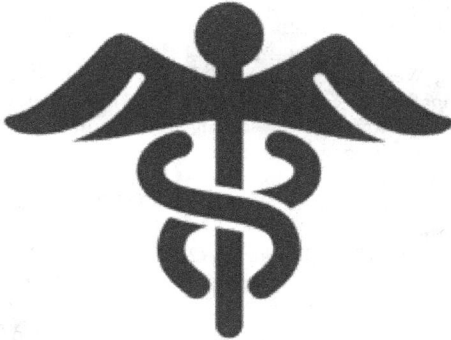

Beacons of Hope

Our path through the mental health system's various crises has led us here. To the current and hopeful future state, where money and problem solvers unite.

Seeds are being sown, and a forest of improvement is in view. Let's review.

Researching the future

During my residency, I was instructing a group of medical students about the importance of psychiatry. I shared that while we enjoy a strong understanding today of the various organs in our body, the brain eludes us still. To any early 1990's girls in the audience, I remind you of the ditty from the teen sensation film *The Babysitter's Club* where the sitters are helping Claudia pass her science test in summer school: "the brain, the brain, the center of the chain."

So, as we move forward with curing the ailment of a broken system, if the brain is the center of the chain, or more precisely for my argument, the center of the spoke, and all healthcare and societal success surrounds the mental health spoke, if we take care of the brain, the wheels can start turning.

Perhaps no one is drafting the future of behavioral health more directly than those involving themselves with research of the brain. Some of the knowledge coming to light as a result of these efforts is astounding.

A doctor's medical education is never really complete. I keep abreast of as much medical research being published as I can. Research of the brain is uncovering astonishing new knowledge all the time, and doctors are sitting in rapt attention like moviegoers at the theater. Some of these findings, of course, may not overly impress the general public; for instance, in 2021, the CDC released a report showing that adults with anxiety or a depressive disorder had increased during the COVID-19 pandemic(Anjel

Vahratian, Stephen J. Blumberg, Emily P. Terlizzi, & Jeannine S. Schiller, 2021). Although that's not a headline that will surprise most people, the scientific breakdown of the increase across demographics can be fascinating.

The research coming down the pike that is the most riveting to me, as a psychiatrist, is that geared towards better understanding our mental health from a biological standpoint. The mental health impacts of physical ailments such as inflammation, gastrointestinal issues, and of course, serotonin deficits, are becoming better understood every day. Psilocybin (yes, the active ingredient in psychoactive mushrooms) is even looking promising as a treatment, or even a cure, for depression. Our once-traditional, simple view of serotonin and depression is expanding rapidly, and research is to thank for this.

Research can surprise you as effectively as any well-written drama. Years ago, I opened a journal to read about a study that had just been completed in Dallas, Texas. It showed that the psychiatric emergency room experienced a statistically significant increase in suicide attempts among women during the spring months (Jeon-Slaughter et al., 2016). The cause? The authors weren't sure, but their best guess: *pollen*. I remember at the time I literally laughed out loud. Pollen! But I managed to keep reading. What these researchers, as well as other studies, have found is that yes, the physical strain of pollen allergies, and related allergies, causes distress to the person, aggravating existing psychological issues and potentially leading to self-harm. But more importantly, inflammation from these allergies contributes to, essentially, an "inflammation storm" in the brain. This causes a shift from "happy" chemicals to toxic chemicals, yielding stressed moods and impulsive behavior. Put another way: allergies may be literally changing our brain chemistry.

Serotonin and Headlines

We as a modern society must recognize our collective and personal responsibility to steer ourselves towards more constructive conversations around mental health. In July of 2022, a review of existing evidence was published in *Molecular Psychiatry* titled "The serotonin theory of depression: a systematic umbrella review of the evidence." (Moncrieff et al., 2022). This review, based out of University College London, was an important brick in the wall of our understanding of depression and its complex relationship with neurotransmitters. Certain popular science outlets thought it was more than that, however; they believed this study called into question the existence of *any* relationship between the neurotransmitter serotonin and clinical depression. Colorful headlines exploded into public view, such as this headline from SciTechDaily: "Scientists Find No Evidence That Depression Is Caused by "Chemical Imbalance" or Low Serotonin Levels." (University College of London, 2022). Or this eye-popping headline from *The Wire Science*: "Depression: New Study Hammers a Nail into the Serotonin Model Coffin." (Datta, 2022). Or this headline from New Scientist: "No link between depression and serotonin, finds major analysis." (Wild, 2022). Even mainstream news got into the act, with *The Guardian* posting this only marginally more restrained headline: "Little evidence that chemical imbalance causes depression, UCL scientists find." (Gregory, 2022). It's only after a half-dozen breathless paragraphs proclaiming the disintegration of the serotonin model of depression that we see a note about "other experts" exhorting people not to stop taking their antidepressant medication. In the Guardian article, a reasonable quote from Dr. Michael Bloomfield from the University College London explaining why people should take these colorful conclusions about the review with a healthy skepticism is buried at the bottom of the article: "Many of us know that taking paracetamol can be helpful for headaches, and I don't think anyone believes that headaches are caused by not enough paracetamol in the brain. The same logic applies to depression and medicines used to treat depression."

The truth is, although selective serotonin reuptake inhibitors (SSRIs) alleviate the symptoms of depression, a lack of serotonin is most likely not the original cause of most depression cases. Psychiatrists have long recognized the causes of depression are multifaceted and dynamic, and lot of research (of mostly the non-headline grabbing kind) has been done in this area establishing models for depression that address this complexity. Psychiatrists take all this research into account when they're considering options for treatment, including SSRIs.

As the most sensational possible narrative took hold for the media cycle, I saw many of my peers in the psychiatric community troubled and even upset by the spin and the lack of context. It seemed irresponsible to drop the suggestion that our most-prescribed medications for depression and anxiety were not having any impact and then simply walk away from the outcry. Weren't these outlets concerned these headlines could undermine the trust between psychiatrists and patients? Were readers likely to take away from this article that the serotonin theory of depression was only one model of depression among many in modern psychiatry? Probably not, on both counts. Did this kind of reporting create a danger that people taking antidepressants for depression and anxiety would see these headlines, assume their medication wasn't working, and stop taking it? I think it's very possible that danger did exist, and still does.

988

A huge milestone occurred recently. On July 16 of 2022, our nation launched the 988 Suicide & Crisis Hotline. This hotline is an expanded version of the pre-existing National Suicide and Crisis Lifeline, with a shorter (and easier to remember) number to dial: 988. This was applauded and strongly supported by mental health professionals, among many others around the country. The act which authorized the new 988 number and expanded call network even received bipartisan support in Congress, being passed by voice vote in both houses (Congress.Gov).

How often does *that* happen?

And yet, the future of this valuable resource is not secure. It's an all too familiar question—where's the money? When former president Donald Trump backed the plan for the new suicide lifeline, the initial funding support of $400 million was allocated for expanding existing Crisis Hotline call centers and improving infrastructure to include texting. But this was a one-time expenditure; sustaining those call centers is the responsibility of the states. At the time of this chapter being written, only 4 states opted to add a fee to phone bills, which, fun fact, is most commonly how states get funding for the 911 number. Others are relying on grants and, in one case as reported by *The New York Times*, GoFundMe (Eder, 2022).

The efficacy of the program is not in doubt. *The New York Times* addressed many concerns in the same article, which was published just a few days prior to launch. 80% of calls to the crisis hotline are resolved. Furthermore, since the 988 launch, the number of calls has increased dramatically. In January of 2023, the Suicide & Crisis Hotline saw 384,071 calls (excluding those calls offered to the Veterans Crisis Line), which was 189,102 more calls than in January of 2022. That's an increase of 57%. Other metrics which have received greater focus since the 988 launch see even more impressive metrics: chats answered have increased 264%, and texts answered have increased an incredible 1608% (Substance Abuse and Mental Health Services Administration).

The 988 program has been so successful, there are already talks about further expanding the program. What is being posed as the "vision for 988" is that mobile crisis teams or mental health triage centers will be available and utilized for those patients who continue to be in crisis during the call to the hotline. Imagine if a mobile team could be dispatched to aid someone experiencing a mental health episode, just like an ambulance for someone having a physical health emergency! Currently, we can only pull from police resources when someone is in need of direct intervention. But who is going to fund those mobile crisis teams or triage centers? That is a question that may have to wait for an answer. States are still finding their footing in the ongoing battle to find funding for the 988 hotline.

My hope for 988 is that it continues to exist as a valuable resource for anyone struggling with an acute mental health situation. But my fear is that the house was built without a foundation. I hope I'm wrong.

Corporate Healthcare

The current landscape sees hospitals sporting names of saints like Saint Joseph or Saint Francis, and psychiatric inpatient facilities with nature-themed appellations like Maple Shade or Twin Oaks. But this may change in the years to come. Instead, we may see facilities flying corporate banners instead of religious or naturalistic ones.

Let's talk about Amazon, once the plucky little-bookseller-that-could that's become a global behemoth. Amazon's annual net income for 2021 was $33 billion (MacroTrends).

Thirty-three billion!

Or, let's look at a company that's smaller but has more of a connection to the healthcare industry: CVS, the largest pharmaceutical retail chain in the United States. In 2021, their net income was $7.91 billion.

Why is this relevant?

In American healthcare's current financial climate, where hospital systems struggle to stay afloat and still deliver quality care, we may have no choice but to look at these giant and well-funded companies to take more of a lead role. If we know addressing mental health care improves overall health and reduces other costs (and we do, but more on that in a minute), then maybe these companies, who have a thicker wallet, can take the frontline approach to helping the mental health crisis, and save healthcare costs down the road.

But why would Amazon or CVS do this? Because frankly, it could be profitable for them. A large enough corporation can handle a large up-front capitalization that standing hospital systems just hanging on simply can't. And with more people becoming mentally healthy, the system financially stabilizes. It is becoming more apparent that if the mental health of employees is addressed, there is an actual return on investment, to the tune of $4 for every $1 spent (National Security Council, 2021).

In November 2022, Amazon launched its own online telehealth clinic. This service connects customers to third party doctors and doles out prescriptions for common ailments (Palmer, 2022). The effort appears to be bearing fruit for the company; in January of 2023, Amazon added an "RxPass" subscription service for generic prescriptions (Ravindranath, 2023). Many might recoil at the idea of a private corporation watching over the gateway to their medicine. But with our care providers straining to make ends meet, and our government deadlocked on how to rectify the situation, what other options are on the table? Can we afford not to at least allow the experiment?

If these experiments in healthcare service models are successful, imagine what they might mean in the future. Imagine a city, population nearing 1 million people. The city has 3 or 4 main hospital systems. Each hospital system has a main hospital campus with an emergency room. Each hospital system also has a psychiatric inpatient hospital, as well as several satellite clinics. Supporting these hospital systems are the Amazon- or CVS-brand mobile psychiatric units and psychiatric emergency rooms. Staffed by psychiatrists, APCs[1], and therapists, the mobile units not only respond as psychiatric emergency vehicles to mental health calls reaching out to 911 or potentially 988, as discussed above, but also liaison with the community hospitals, ensuring-near immediate response to those in crisis.

Is it ideal that these services would be offered by private corporations, instead of dedicated non-profit or public entities? Probably not, but our industry is hitting a breaking point and, speaking as a professional watching the mental health crisis unfold from the front row, I can tell you that we're running out of time to find a better solution.

As a resident in training, I remember a call I received one day from a reputable cardiologist whose clinic was on the same hospital grounds as the psychiatry consult and liaison service line. Despite this doctor's impressive expertise in his field, he found himself in a situation where he did not know how to proceed: an acutely suicidal patient. The doctor knew he wanted to get his patient to an emergency room, located only a short distance away from the grounds.

---

[1] Advanced Practice Clinicians

His difficulty was making sure the patient got there safely. He did not want a police presence to startle the patient, and he worried that calling 911 or EMSA (Emergency Medical Services Authority) would be excessive and costly. He asked if a family member could escort the patient to the emergency room.

I advised that EMSA is usually notified in these situations to ensure the patient safely arrives in the emergency room. Though I still believe that was the right call, I could not help thinking about the large price tag associated with any ambulance call.

So, am I suggesting the Amazon Prime gray sprinter van arrives to the clinic to address this patient's needs? No. But try replicating this scenario off a hospital campus, in an isolated clinic or perhaps a general rural setting, where options may be limited. Could care brought to the patient by these sources eliminate a crisis that would otherwise go unattended to?

These efforts have already begun. Companies across the country are trying to fill this middle ground between the home, clinic, emergency room, and hospital. Filling the gaps of care between these settings to ensure urgently-needed care is delivered, and with an available treatment plan for continued care after crisis, is key to making these systems work in the future.

This Isn't Working

Anjel Vahratian, P., Stephen J. Blumberg, P., Emily P. Terlizzi, M., & Jeannine S. Schiller, M. (2021). Symptoms of Anxiety or Depressive Disorder and Use of Mental Health Care Among Adults During the COVID-19 Pandemic — United States, August 2020–February 2021. *Morbidity and Mortality Weekly Report*, 70(13);490–494.

Congress.Gov. *S.2661 - National Suicide Hotline Designation Act of 2020*. Retrieved from https://www.congress.gov/bill/116th-congress/senate-bill/2661/actions.

Datta, S. (2022). Depression: New Study Hammers a Nail into the Serotonin Model Coffin. *The Wire Science*. Retrieved from https://science.thewire.in/the-sciences/serotonin-model-depression-repeal/

Eder, A. O. a. S. (Producer). (2022, July 15). The U.S. Has a New Crisis Hotline: 988. Is It Prepared for a Surge in Calls? *The New York Times*. Retrieved from https://www.nytimes.com/2022/07/15/us/988-mental-health-lifeline.html

Gregory, A. (2022). Little evidence that chemical imbalance causes depression, UCL scientists find. *The Guardian*. Retrieved from https://www.theguardian.com/society/2022/jul/20/scientists-question-widespread-use-of-antidepressants-after-survey-on-serotonin

Jeon-Slaughter, H., Claassen, C. A., Khan, D. A., Mihalakos, P., Lee, K. B., & Brown, E. S. (2016). Temporal Association Between Nonfatal Self-Directed Violence and Tree and Grass Pollen Counts. *Journal of Clinical Psychiatry*.

MacroTrends. Amazon Net Income 2010-2022. Retrieved from https://www.macrotrends.net/stocks/charts/AMZN/amazon/net-income

Moncrieff, J., Cooper, R. E., Stockmann, T., Amendola, S., Hengartner, M. P., & Horowitz, M. A. (2022). The serotonin theory of depression: a systematic umbrella review of the evidence. *Molecular Psychiatry*.

National Security Council (Producer). (2021, May 13). New Mental Health Cost Calculator Shows Why Investing in Mental Health is Good for Business. *Information sheet. www. who. int/mental_health/management/info_sheet. pdf.* Retrieved from https://www.nsc.org/newsroom/new-mental-health-cost-calculator-demonstrates-why

Palmer, K. (Producer). (2022, November 15). Amazon jumps into direct-to-consumer telehealth, launching a rival to Ro and Hims. *Stat News*. Retrieved from https://www.statnews.com/2022/11/15/amazon-clinic-

telehealth-ro-
hims/?utm_campaign=health_tech&utm_medium=email&_
hsmi=242967719&_hsenc=p2ANqtz-
9IV79zIOI2tLYTz4y8Mf8B92TTogfyLWiX32lpKkZLgQljZ
Zp1KrdWupBaWS6i4JsXvL9HHX3D9WoovOtwVpDk9zw
uzkey6RI4xBHF1bavQ0Fdjs

Ravindranath, M. (Producer). (2023, January 24). Amazon Prime for your prescriptions, virtual care during pregnancy, & AI for mental health. *Stat News*. Retrieved from https://www.statnews.com/2023/01/24/amazon-pharmacy-health-tech-pregnancy/

Substance Abuse and Mental Health Services Administration. 988 Lifeline Performance Metrics. *SAMHSA Substance Abuse and Mental Health Services Administration*. Retrieved from https://www.samhsa.gov/find-help/988/performance-metrics

University College of London. (2022). Scientists Find No Evidence That Depression Is Caused by "Chemical Imbalance" or Low Serotonin Levels. *SciTechDaily*. Retrieved from https://scitechdaily.com/scientists-find-no-evidence-that-depression-is-caused-by-chemical-imbalance-or-low-serotonin-levels/

Wild, S. (2022). No link between depression and serotonin, finds major analysis. *New Scientist*. Retrieved from https://www.newscientist.com/article/2328700-no-link-between-depression-and-serotonin-finds-major-analysis/

This Isn't Working

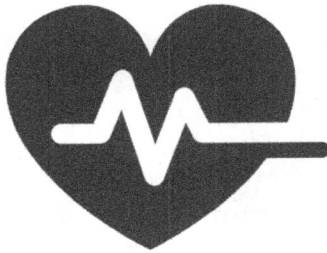

Conclusion

My hope is the preceding chapters have allowed you to peek behind the curtain of mental health and the health industry in general, but also, invited curiosity and more questions about the mental health crisis in our world.

Together, we have attempted to "lift the veil" into the world of mental health and the specific trials and tribulations threatening this important system. We've scaled some daunting data and even examined the cases based on real-life patients. I've tried to accurately convey the whole picture of a situation that I honestly believe is dire. But what I don't want to do is leave you feeling the situation is actually without hope of improvement.

As a psychiatrist, I feel it healthy and necessary to leave you on a good note, with hope, and some evidence that the mental health system still does good work.

I have seen patients from nearly all walks of life. I have treated people who live on the streets, people who were released from jail hours prior, people who were intoxicated, suicidal, or even homicidal. I've seen people who looked on the outside like they had it all, while secretly they were in a horrible struggle. I've sat with a woman in the deepest throes of grief on what should have been her happiest day, after delivering a stillborn baby.

And what I know, after treating so many different cases, is that people can and do get better. You can go from barely getting out of bed to becoming employed and finding that social life you may have thought was unreachable. I have been there for those cases. If you're a new mother, you can struggle through that postpartum depression to find joy and meaning in learning the role of motherhood. I've seen those, too. Even at the end of your life, you can find peace and happiness. I've been there for this as well. I bid farewell to a most dear patient who struggled with depression his whole life. As the cancer took over and his care was assumed by hospice, in our final meeting he told me the last year and a half of our meetings were the happiest he had been, despite a very aggressive and painful cancer.

Am I the best psychiatrist? No. For me, being a psychiatrist has meant painfully learning my limits, again and again, both as a doctor and as a human being. And some of the most important things I've learned have been the simplest. A common thread I have seen in my patients and in our society is a need to be heard, to be loved, and to be seen.

With the last patient mentioned, who I'll call John, I found my job was mostly to listen. I also found mutual interests. I disclosed, when I felt it therapeutic. When things turned for the worse, I held his hand in the hospital. Having known him for a year at that point, I felt confident his hand had not been held in a very long time, maybe since the dissolution of his marriage, decades prior. John was a sweet, friendly man, a favorite patient of the hospital, but his life had been very lonely. I will never forget his face as I sat there, with him and his brother, the only family he had. Even this connection lived 1300 miles away. My patient looked at me with tears in his eyes. He had learned nothing was working and the tumor was becoming bigger. The finality of life was imminent. Soon he would be moved to a critical care facility, where he would spend the last days of his life. He told me he was scared, a feeling he had always tried to fight off during our conversations. I grabbed his hand tighter and told him I was here. It was a reminder that in that moment, he was seen, that he mattered to someone. He squeezed my hand, took a deep breath, closed his eyes to rest.

So many of our conflicts in society stem from this need for connection. Look at the "groupaphilia" in our society. Yes, I made up that word. Look at the deep-seated need in individuals to find a group and an identity with the hopes they will be seen, heard, cared for, and loved. This manifests in countless ways: from gang affiliations to drama clubs, and from mahjong groups to the endless corridors of social media. Obviously, some of these groups are more constructive than others. But why do humans have this tendency to group up at all? It is an innate need to feel the support of others, to feel psychologically cared for. Often, we are specifically seeking to be cared for in those ways in which we were not in our younger, formative years.

Freud, and the countless others who followed him, studied the behaviors of humans intensely and intimately. He concluded, even working from different schools of psychological theory, that people *suffer* from their emotions, and to erase that suffering takes work. It is with great intent, purpose, and might that one can find happiness in this world. But as we have seen, those who seek assistance in repairing their mental health may face adversity, roadblocks, and dead ends.

We as a modern society must recognize our collective and personal responsibility to steer ourselves towards more constructive conversations around mental health.

Our growing mental health crisis is being called "the next pandemic" in outlets like *The Wall Street Journal (Henninger, 2022)* and Gallup.com (Clifton, 2021). I recognize a problem that big cannot be solved in these pages, or a new law, or improvements in science reporting, or a merging of companies, or even a new suicide lifeline number. But my hope is the conversation around this system that facilitates my life's work doesn't stop. We need for the thinkers to get together and recognize the speed bumps, the roadblocks, the dead ends, to examine them and create a path to navigate it for those who need it. If they won't, if we don't spur the conversation, the people who will most suffer will be those ones who struggle daily, the ones who are desperate yet unsure of where to start, and those who may not win the fight on their own. To witness the transformation in someone who feels their life is now worth living because of work we've done in my office is an overwhelming privilege and my life's work. The intimacy and trust that must exist to help someone achieve a new willingness to live each day does not come easily, and so it is that this much larger problem's solution will not come easily. But mental health care services are too critically important not to put that work in.

Look at any area in our lives and see how mental health care impacts that area. From the womb to the end of life, the psychological string that connects all parts of our society is frazzled and tender. In mental health care, the care provided may not help the patient to breathe better, eradicate their cancer, or remove some physical ailment. But it does help the patient to fully live better.

In a climate of distrust, media mayhem, isolation, financial uncertainty, and invisible personal distress, where self-help books abound, articles and social media posts sensationally promising the "key to happiness" are numberless. Meanwhile, start-up health clinics soaking the nation in stimulants and Xanax thrived overnight. It would be natural to pull *down* the veil separating us from these causes, ignore the issues, and find another more tangible problem in society to fix. But as a mental health weatherwoman of sorts, standing in front of a green screen, motioning to the incoming storm with headlines of depression, anxiety, and the overall general sense that people in this world are struggling to find happiness, I ask that we continue to lift that veil with all our might as our lives depend on it.

Clifton, J. (Producer). (2021, December 3). "The Next Global Pandemic: Mental Health". *Gallup*. Retrieved from https://www.gallup.com/workplace/357710/next-global-pandemic-mental-health.aspx#:~:text=What%20if%20the%20next%20global,reached%20record%20highs%20in%202020.

Henninger, D. (Producer). (2022, May 18). "The Next Pandemic: Mental Illness". *The Wall Street Journal*.

This Isn't Working

ABOUT THE AUTHOR

Dr. Natalie Kurkjian is a practicing board-certified psychiatrist with a clinical focus on patients with oncologic disease or dementia. She also serves as the medical director of Behavioral Health in her health system. She has a strong interest in helping patients understand and navigate their own healthcare.